KITCHEN PHARMACY

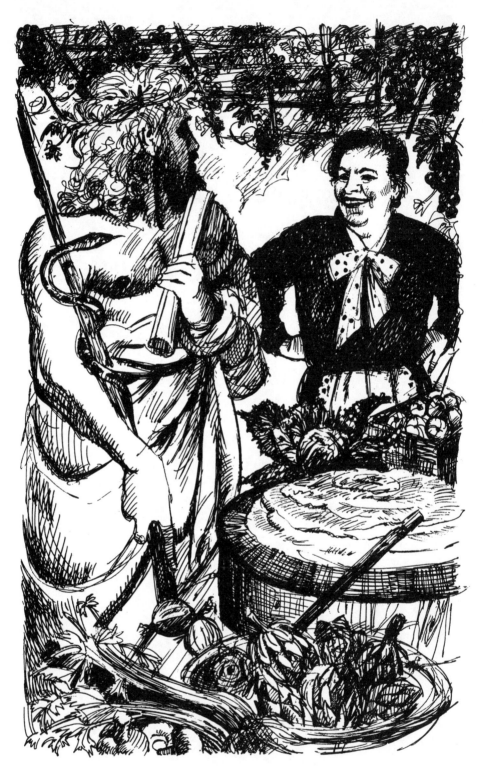

A polenta feast for Asclepius

KITCHEN PHARMACY

A Book of Healing Remedies for Everyone

ROSE ELLIOT AND CARLO DE PAOLI

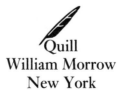

Quill
William Morrow
New York

Library of Congress Cataloging-in-Publication Data

Elliot, Rose.
   Kitchen pharmacy : a book of healing remedies for everyone / Rose Elliot and Carlo De Paoli.
     p. cm.
   Includes bibliographical references (p.   ) and index.
   ISBN 0-688-12111-X
   1. Diet therapy. 2. Materia medica, Vegetable. 3. Medicine, Popular. 4. Herbs—Therapeutic use. I. De Paoli, Carlo. II. Title.
RM216.E52 1992
615'.321—dc20   92-20651
                                       CIP

Printed in the United States of America

First Quill Edition

1 2 3 4 5 6 7 8 9 10

BOOK DESIGN BY RONALD CLARK

Contents

Acknowledgements

We should like to express our special appreciation and love to Ian and Marjory Chapman for their belief in and enthusiasm for this project from the very beginning; to Robert Elliot for support, patience and wisdom throughout; to André Durand for his superb drawings; to Ron Clark for his invaluable input in the design; to Greg Hill, David North and Christine Hoy for their wonderful backing, enthusiasm and expertise as ever; to Barbara Levy, literary agent, for support at all stages; to Kelly Davis for her usual brilliant editing and for being such a pleasure to work with. In addition, grateful thanks to Gilean Reid Walker for calligraphy; to Fiona Edwards for botanical advice; to Yvonne Holland for help with the proofs; to Kate Truman and Jackie Dobbyn for proofreading; to Barbara James for the indexes.

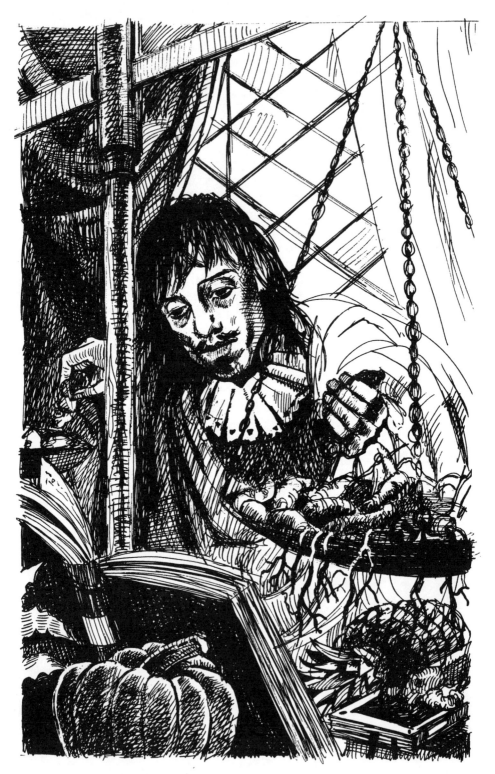

Nicholas Culpeper (1616–54) studying the medicinal properties of herbs

Introduction

Kitchen Pharmacy is primarily a book of self-help. We aim to describe, simply and clearly, how anyone can use widely available natural ingredients to help them to keep well, to treat minor ailments, and to assist the healing process. The book blends ideas from both Eastern and Western natural medicine, explaining them in a straightforward, practical way. It also looks at the role of our minds and emotions in our total health and how we can help the healing process by adopting a harmonious and energy-raising lifestyle.

Many of us would find it useful to know what soup to give to soothe a cough or sore chest; to be able to ease a sore throat with an effective gargle made from everyday kitchen ingredients; or to bring relief to burning indigestion with the right choice of herb tea or a simple massage with essential oils. In fact it's only in the last few decades that we have got out of the habit of treating ourselves with plants and herbs and have come to rely so much on doctors. If you think about it, you'll probably find that you already use quite a few natural remedies without even realising it – lemon and honey for a sore throat, for instance, prunes for constipation, or vinegar to treat a wasp sting.

Kitchen Pharmacy describes the contribution which diets and remedies prepared from the herbs and spices, grains, fruits, vegetables and flowers of the kitchen can make to health and healing. The nutritional suggestions and remedies are intended to complement, not replace, diagnosis and treatment by a medical practitioner, or other qualified healer or therapist. Any major ailment or acute condition requires prompt medical attention *before* you consider any type of self-treatment. Once the immediate crisis has passed, natural remedies can be highly effective as aids to long-term healing. They can also be of great benefit in helping to prevent a relatively minor ailment from developing into a more serious condition.

To put these natural remedies in context, the book starts with a brief review of the history of natural healing; then looks at the Chinese view of energy and its two manifestations, yin and yang.

The core of the book, the 'Remedies' chapter, describes all the herbs, vegetables and fruits and their qualities and roles in the healing process. It tells you how to prepare them and includes many delicious healing recipes. This is followed by a complementary 'Ailments' chapter which advises you on how to treat specific ailments. Finally there is a chapter on other aids to healing, such as exercise, meditation and affirmations.

We have tried to make the book as helpful as possible, so that you find it easy to refer to. The basic principles of self-treatment are really quite simple. Once you have got to know them we hope your copy of *Kitchen Pharmacy* will soon become a trusted friend, there to be consulted at all times.

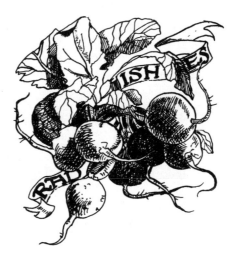

How to Use This Book

If you begin by reading the chapter on 'Diagnosis and Diets' you will gain an overview of the main principles of kitchen pharmacy, and you may recognise your symptoms under one or more of the Basic Conditions. You can then look up the recommended herbs and foods in the 'Remedies' chapter. Alternatively you may wish to refer to the relevant section in 'Ailments' to see whether the symptoms described under a specific illness sound familiar. If you have already identified your ailment you may prefer to consult the Index which will refer you to all the relevant remedies.

To make it easier for you to find the information you need, we have printed references to section headings in bold type and references to particular ailments and recipes in capital letters.

You may also find it useful to refer to the chart on page 277 which lists all the herbs, spices and foods under their main qualities. If you have a hot condition, for example, you can see at a glance which foods are cooling and which foods will exacerbate the problem.

Using the Remedies

Most of the foods, herbs, teas and tinctures mentioned in this book are widely available at supermarkets or healthfood shops. For the more unusual ones, you may need to contact one of the specialist suppliers listed in your Yellow Pages.

In the main text we generally refer to the remedies by their common names. However, some of them may be marketed under their Latin names. (For instance, marigold ointment is usually sold as calendula ointment.) If you need to find out the Latin name of a particular plant or herb you can look it up in the list on page 275.

When using any of the remedies, do follow the guidelines given on pages 41–5; always start with the smallest suggested dosage and increase this gradually. Do not continue the treatment for longer than the recommended period and *always* get the advice of a qualified medical practitioner if symptoms persist, or if you are in doubt.

You will find instructions for making infusions, teas, decoctions, tinctures, compresses and poultices, and using essential oils in baths and massages, on pages 41–5.

When using any of the recipes given in the 'Remedies' chapter, do bear in mind that you may need to adapt them to your particular condition. For instance, if you have a hot condition you will need to omit or replace any hot spices. The chart on page 277 will give you ideas for more cooling flavourings. Likewise, if you suffer from oedema (fluid retention) you will need to avoid salt.

A NOTE ABOUT MEASUREMENTS

In all the recipes and remedies:

1 teaspoon   =   5 ml
1 tablespoon   = 15 ml
'a saucer'   = about 85 ml/3 fl oz
'a cup/cupful' = about 150 ml/5 fl oz (i.e. an ordinary kitchen teacup rather than a standard cup measurement)

Treating Children

The advice given in this book can be used for treating children as well as adults. Look up their symptoms in the usual way, and naturally always seek medical advice if you have any cause for concern. In any case, it's better to get medical advice if the child is under 3.

When treating children, use tinctures and essential oils as described on pages 43–5, reducing the dosages according to the age of the child as follows:

3–4 years: 3–4 drops of tincture twice a day
6–12 years: 7 drops of tincture twice a day
12–16 years: 15 drops of tincture twice a day

Essential oils should be well-diluted for children, and never put into the bath without being mixed with a little oil or milk first. For massage, use 5–10 drops to 100 ml/3½ fl oz base oil and then mix again with 100 ml base oil, for children under 6, increasing the amount of essential oil gradually according to age.

KITCHEN
PHARMACY

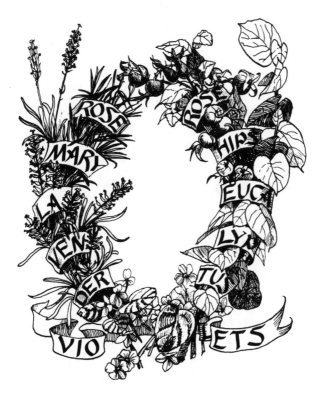

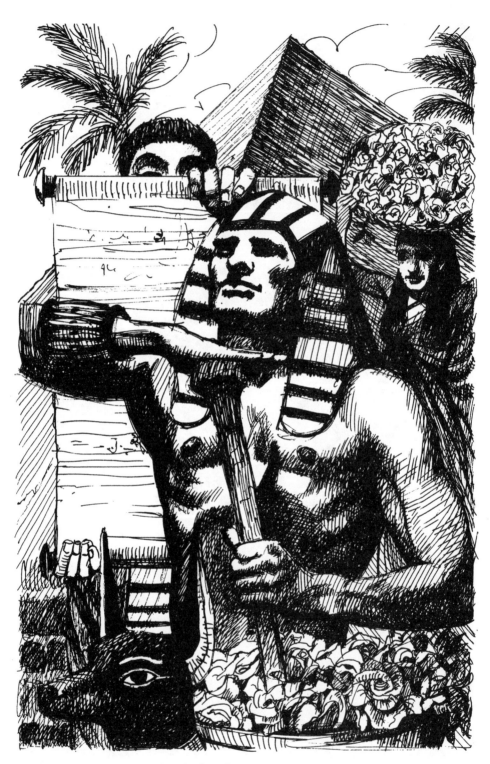

Maceration of roses, Egypt 1300 BC

1

The Ancient Tradition of Natural Healing

❧

The tradition of kitchen pharmacy is both ancient and universal. It has evolved over the centuries through the observation by ordinary men and women, and physicians, of the effect on the body of common ingredients. For example, remains of medicinal herbs, some still used today, were excavated in 1960 in northern Iraq in a burial ground dating back 50,000 years. From such early beginnings, traditional systems of healing developed.

Whilst each country had its own particular approach, and some unique remedies, many other plants and treatments were common to several. Information was exchanged by early travellers and sometimes a country would borrow the food and medicines of another for a number of centuries. Myrrh, for example, was first used in Egypt, then travelled to Greece and Arabia, and from there to India and thence to China. It is interesting that even where there was no contact, ingredients were often independently given exactly the same classification by different cultures. Garlic, for instance, was universally classified as being anti-septic and expectoral, liquorice as anti-inflammatory and digestive, and fennel as aromatic and wind-expelling.

The Egyptians had one of the oldest traditions of kitchen pharmacy dating back perhaps as far as 3000 BC. In their mythology, the gods Isis, Horus and Osiris were the dispensers of medical knowledge. The Ebers papers, important 1500 BC Egyptian manuscripts recording much earlier information, mention as many as 500 medicinal substances, many of them culinary items still widely used today, such as mint and cinnamon. Homer described Egypt as a 'fertile land that produces an abundance of medicinal drugs, some as remedies, others as perfumes; country of the wisest physicians in the whole world.' Most Egyptian temples had laboratories where plant medicines and essential oils were produced. We find mention of this in their textbooks, and in the hieroglyphics on their pyramids and tombs.

Later, medical authors like Pliny, Galen, Dioscorides and Theophras-tus record renowned Egyptian perfumes which were sold worldwide at

15

high prices. Dioscorides wrote in his *De Materia Medica* in the first century AD about a mixture, sacred to the gods, which the Egyptians had been using for many centuries. It was called kyphi and it contained, among other things, juniper berries, cypress seeds, myrrh, cinnamon, cardamom, calamus, raisins, old wine and honey. It was used as a blood purifier, a mood uplifter, a remedy for colds and asthma, a tonic and even a perfume. During the preparation of kyphi, priests read the formula and mode of preparation from sacred texts. As we know, their understanding of medicinal plants and oils enabled the Egyptians to preserve mummified bodies for thousands of years, eliminating the decomposing and putrefying action of micro-organisms.

The knowledge of the Egyptians penetrated civilisations in Babylonia and Assyria, and influenced later ones in Arabia, Greece and Rome. Through these countries, valuable information was disseminated through the rest of Europe, India and China. Greece was also the birthplace of two prominent exponents of Western traditional medicine: Pythagoras (600–500 BC), acclaimed philosopher, physician and teacher of natural sciences; and Hippocrates (460–377 BC) who graduated from the Pythagorean school. Hippocrates travelled widely, studying the medicinal properties of plants and food and gathering such a body of knowledge that he became known as 'the father of medicine'. During the 430 BC plague in Athens, Hippocrates instructed his assistants to brew aromatic herbs and spices such as thyme, sage and marjoram on all the street corners. Modern scientific research has shown these herbs to have a strong anti-microbial action.

India developed a highly evolved system of medicine which, though mainly based on herbs, also included many minerals and (like that of the Egyptians) surgery. The *Susruta Samitha*, thought to date from 50 AD, describes 500 remedies and 125 surgical instruments.

However, perhaps the greatest contribution to modern holistic medicine and kitchen pharmacy has come from China. The Chinese system of healing is one of the oldest and has influenced the whole of Far Eastern Asia. Herbal prescriptions for various illnesses have been found, written on carapaces and bones, dating back to the Yin dynasty (1500 BC). During the Zhou dynasty (1100 BC), one of the names for medicine was *yao*, which means 'the grasses which cure disease'. In Chinese Tao philosophy, medicine became part of a spiritual way of life in which the balancing of the opposites, yin and yang, brought well-being and peace of mind. Lao-Tsu (500 BC), founder of Taoism, described this condition of universal harmony in the *Tao Te Ching*: 'Man follows the ways of earth, earth follows the ways of Heaven, Heaven follows the ways of Tao, Tao follows its own nature.'

When the *Canon of Medicine* or *Huangoi Neijin*, believed to have been written by the mythical Yellow Emperor, appeared around 300–400 BC, medicine and philosophy were fully integrated. This text explains both the theory of yin and yang, and the circulation of the chi, or energy. When many members of his family died from fever, a scholar called Zhang Zhongjing devoted his life to the study of medicine and, around 200 BC, wrote the *Discussions of Fevers*. One of the remedies in this book is 'cinnamon sap soup' which contains cinnamon, ginger, dates, liquorice and Chinese peony, and is still widely used in China as a folk medicine for colds and flu.

In the West, with the advent of chemical medicine, traditional kitchen medicine slowly started to decline from the sixteenth century onwards. Meanwhile, traditional Chinese medicine continued to flourish, enjoying great patronage from the ruling classes. After the Communist takeover in China the government invested a great deal in scientific research on both traditional and modern medicine. Thousands of experiments on the properties of natural remedies have been carried out and meticulously recorded since the early 1950s, confirming their value and enabling them to be used very effectively. (We refer to some of these experiments under particular remedies in this book.)

Although traditional Chinese medicine has been the subject of considerable scientific research, its approach is still firmly rooted in ancient classics such as the much-celebrated *Grand Materia Medica* of Li Shi-Zhen (1500 AD) which describes 1892 substances, of which 1173 are derived from plants. In 1977 the Jiang Su College of New Medicine, after 25 years of research, published the *Encyclopaedia of Traditional Medicinal Substances* listing the therapeutic properties of over 5000 substances.

Galen of Pergamum (130–201 AD), one of the great forefathers of Western traditional medicine, was thoroughly acquainted with the work of Pythagoras, Hippocrates, Dioscorides and the worshippers of Asclepius, god of health. His greatest contribution was to categorise each herb as hot, cold, moist or dry, and also to specify the degree to which these qualities were present. This approach was in harmony with Indian and Chinese medicine and became the basis for European nature cure and herbalism until the scientific revolution. Galen believed that one had to consider not only the disease from which the patient was suffering, but also his particular energetic imbalance. For instance, if ten patients had stomach ulcers each one would be treated differently according to the energetic imbalance which had created the problem. In contrast, modern medicine would seek to find a cure for all cases of stomach ulcers, irrespective of their causes.

In the meantime, people in the Arab world, inspired by the works of Galen, had been developing their own kitchen pharmacy and herbalism. Owing to their geographical position, they bridged the gap between the European and Egyptian traditions on one side, and the Indian and Chinese on the other. Their channelling of medical information between these civilisations was vital in expanding traditional medicine. In the eleventh century the Arabian physician Avicenna wrote one of the most important Western *materia medica, Al Quanum;* and in the thirteenth century, Al Baitar wrote a medical book which listed 2000 substances, many of which were plants.

The Crusaders and Knights Templar brought much of this information back to Europe, giving further impetus to the work of herbalists. With the advent of Christianity, especially after the eleventh century, the tradition of kitchen pharmacy and nature cure was continued through monks and nuns who studied the medical classics in their monasteries and convents. By the twelfth century, in Europe, as in Arabia and the East, the gardens of kings and religious orders contained many of the main ingredients for kitchen pharmacy and herbal medicine. In his book *De Naturis Rerum*, the Abbot of the Augustines at Cirencester described the ideal nobleman's garden:

> It should be adorned with roses, lilies, turnsole [sunflowers], violets and mandrake; there you should have parsley and cost [chard], and fennel and southernwood and coriander, sage, savory, hyssop etc . . . There should be planted beds with onions, leeks, garlick, pumpkin . . .

Most of these plants were used both for culinary and medicinal purposes.

A great deal of this new knowledge was encapsulated throughout the Middle Ages by the Salernitan school (one of the biggest medieval European schools of natural medicine, based in Salerno, Italy). They made extensive use of spices, such as sage, cloves and thyme, for their antiseptic qualities; mint and fennel for the digestive tract; and watercress against scurvy. Continuing the European tradition, Abbess Hildegard of Bingen (1098–1179), in her book *Liber Simplicis Medicinae* gave detailed descriptions of the curative properties of many spices, plants and foods, and their relationship to moods and spiritual growth. Notable

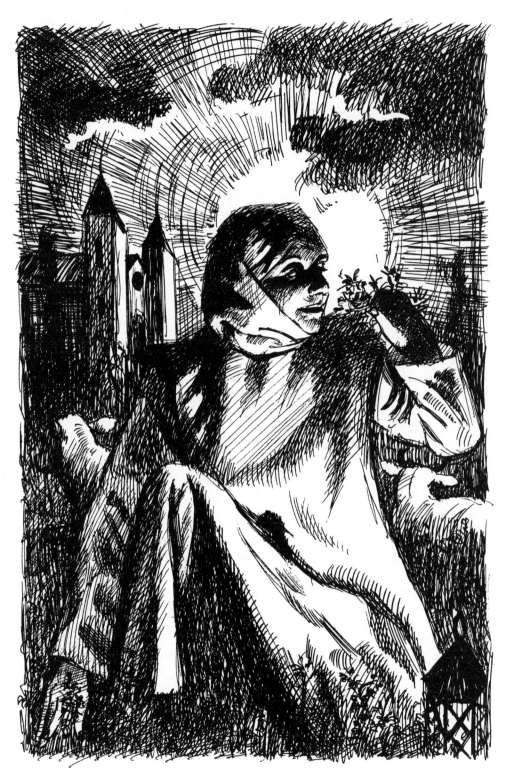

Hildegard of Bingen (1098–1179) gathering herbs by moonlight

English doctors were Nicholas Culpeper (1616–54), who furthered the tradition of Galen, linking plants to the personality in his *Physicall Directory* (1649); and Gerard, author of the *Herbal or General History of Plants*, with 2850 descriptions of plants and 2700 illustrations. In France, the physician Michel de Notradame, also known as Nostradamus (1503–66), used natural ingredients, including rosehips, to make a pill which he administered to people suffering from the plague.

Although much of their traditional knowledge was lost, the Indians of North America contributed greatly to human health and survival with agents like boneset for fevers, and ipecacuanha for bronchitis, as well as an American variety of ginseng which is widely used in China nowadays.

Today, of the Western countries, France has probably made the most important contribution to modern understanding of natural medicine through the work of Cadeac and Meunier 1889–92; and in the 1950s, Prof. L. Binet, Dean of the Faculty of Medicine in Paris; also Leclerc, Dusquesnois and Rène Paris, founder of the International Museum of Herbal Medicine. All followers of natural medicine and kitchen pharmacy are highly indebted to the French doctor, J. Valnet. In the 1950s, while serving as a doctor with the French Army in Indochina, Dr Valnet ran short of disinfectants and used some essential oils to treat wounds and cleanse his premises. He was so impressed with the results that he dedicated his life to the research and promotion of natural medicine. He wrote some of the most important modern books available on kitchen pharmacy. In Italy, Cojola and Rovesti were important modern researchers, and in Germany, Bruer, and Arreo Muller.

Most modern research on herbal remedies simply confirms what has been empirically observed over the centuries. For example, in the past many thousands of sailors used to die unnecessarily of scurvy, although many old schools of medicine recommended fresh vegetables and fruits to protect against it. In the eighteenth century an English naval doctor decided to experiment with this formula and the result was that scurvy was totally eradicated from the Navy. Two hundred years later, researchers discovered vitamin C in fresh fruit and vegetables and showed its efficacy against scurvy.

To quote another example, for centuries onions were known as an aid in diabetes; then, between 1924 and 1934, the researchers Collip and Laurin discovered that onions contained chemicals which had an anti-diabetic action. Vervain, too, had its centuries-old reputation for facilitating childbirth proved recently when a Japanese researcher, Kotoku

Kuwazine, discovered in the plant a powerful activator of uterine contractions. Similarly, scientists have recently found oestrogen-inducing substances in sage, a herb which has always been used for menstrual and menopausal problems. The anti-microbial properties of plants like garlic, thyme and lemon are also being rediscovered. Tests on microbial cultures have shown that these plants can very often kill powerful microbes more quickly and efficiently than chemical remedies.

Nowadays natural practitioners believe that treatment with chemical drugs has serious disadvantages. Most importantly, drugs are made from inorganic substances, whilst the cells of our bodies are organic, as are those of the food we eat. An organic cell is one which can duplicate, grow, eliminate and then perish. Our bodies are not designed to absorb inorganic matter. Substances which we can tolerate in large quantities in their organic form become toxic, even in small doses, when inorganic. For instance, seaweeds contain a great deal of organic iodine which we can easily absorb and benefit from. But taking even the smallest amount of chemical iodine can make us very ill. This is why chemical medicine can be so toxic.

Chemical medicine has two further serious drawbacks. Firstly, when taken in and assimilated by the body, a substance may have a different action from that observed in laboratory tests. Secondly, in its natural form, a medicinal plant may be extremely complex and subtle, containing hundreds of different chemicals. Although one of these might seem to predominate, the main therapeutic effect of the plant occurs because of the interaction of many substances. When one of these is isolated, the delicate balance is upset. For instance, it is well-known that chemical diuretics can be very damaging because they create inflammation in the kidneys and deplete the body's store of potassium. However, dandelion (which is a natural diuretic) does not cause these problems. Along with some very powerful diuretic chemicals, it contains many anti-inflammatory agents, as well as much natural potassium.

Although some chemical drugs are stronger, many natural substances, if properly and judiciously administered, can have a similar, if not more powerful effect, and a much safer one. As we have seen, natural medicine has had a glorious past. If, in modern times, research on natural remedies had received a fraction of the funds which have been put into the pharmaceutical industries, we might now be able to tackle, officially and effectively, many major diseases in a natural way. There are, nevertheless, many remedies which we can safely use ourselves, with excellent results.

21

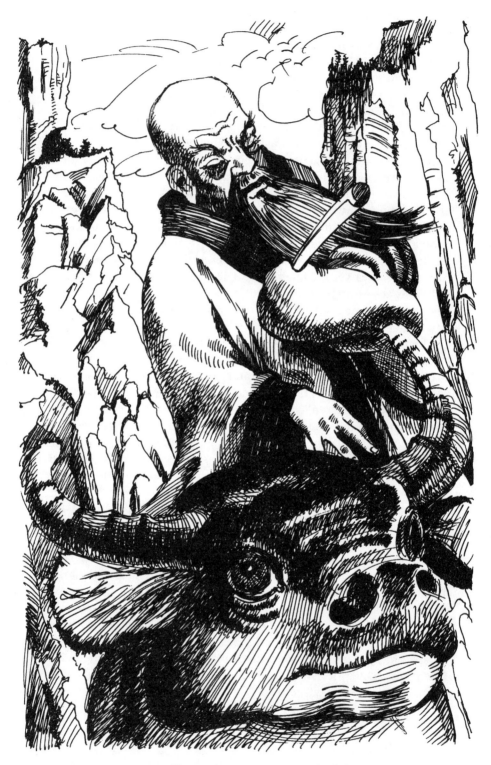

Lao-Tsu travelling to the West on a water-buffalo, 500 BC

2
Diagnosis and Diets

Energy, Foundation of Life

At the heart of traditional Chinese medicine is the belief that all life is an expression of energy. This energy is thought to manifest in different concentrations in the spirit, emotions, mind and body. At the most rarefied level, the ancient Chinese believed, was found the spiritual being, the 'Self', which connects us with the whole of the Universe. Next came slightly denser levels, the emotions, and the mind. Finally, at the bottom of the scale, was the material world, including the physical body and all its organs, which were considered to be the densest expression of energy. So, while in the West these aspects of life were thought of as separate, in the East they were considered as different manifestations of the same thing: energy.

The Chinese even went so far as to link each major organ of the body with an emotion and view them both as manifestations of the same energy (for more on this, see pages 263–9). Imbalances in one level of energy were thought to affect the other levels. This could start at the physical level and work upwards (a physical ailment affecting our mind and emotions) or it could start at the higher levels and work down (an emotion such as fear or worry manifesting on the physical level as illness). Treatment, equally, could be given at either end of the scale; for example, using acupuncture and herbs on the physical body would bring balance to the organs, and the emotions associated with them would also be harmonised. Or healing at the emotional and mental level, with techniques such as counselling, meditation and visualisation, would help to cure ailments in the physical body. This philosophy, which has existed for thousands of years, is now being rediscovered in modern holistic medicine in which the whole person, not just the body, is treated.

Energy is not static; it moves and flows, and in order to do so it needs two poles, as in the positive and negative connections in electricity, so that it can go from one point to another. The Chinese called this phenomenon of energy moving between two poles the polarity of yin and yang, yin being one point and yang being the other. All aspects of life can be defined as being either yin or yang. However, we need to realise that everything is yin in relation to yang, and vice versa. For instance, to give examples from the kitchen, grains are yin in relation to meats, but they are yang in relation to fruits. The chart below gives some more examples.

YIN	YANG
cool/cold	warm/hot
receptive	active
dark	bright
winter	summer
internal	external
earth	sky
soft	hard
flexible	rigid
moist	dry
regeneration	expansion
rest	activity

It is important to understand that yin and yang are interdependent and equally important. If there was only winter, nothing would grow; if there was only summer, plants would burn. Yin transforms itself into yang, and vice versa, as shown in the movement of the seasons from summer to winter, and of day to night, of activity followed by the need for rest. Some books have over-emphasised the positive importance of being yang, describing yin as weak, lazy, slow, sluggish and so on, and yang as strong, positive, bright, and energetic. In fact, in traditional Chinese thought, yin has at times been considered even more vital than yang energy. Without enough yin energy, the body becomes dry, consumed, restless, hot and barren. A person who is more yin in a healthy way can be one who is jovial, relaxed, sympathetic and receptive. Excesses of either yin or yang are harmful; the ideal is to have the two balanced harmoniously, as in the well-known symbol showing two intertwined figures within a circle, one black and one white.

The Basic Conditions

The system of diagnosis described here is a simplified version of the one used in traditional Chinese medicine, which has developed over thousands of years. In this system, the energy level and condition of the patient is analysed both by observation and by taking the pulse. It can take years to master this type of diagnosis, so we can only offer a simple guide to the basic principles here.

According to traditional Chinese medicine, different types of energy imbalance are the root cause of most illnesses. We call these imbalances the basic conditions. These conditions do not necessarily influence every organ in the body; sometimes they might only affect one organ; at other times, more than one. A patient might also be suffering from more than one condition affecting two or more organs.

Don't worry if some of the terms seem strange at first, or if you find it difficult to grasp all the ideas straight away. You will find them expressed again in the chapters on 'Remedies' and 'Ailments'. As you read and use the book you will find that these ideas become very familiar to you and start to make sense as part of a wider picture of the whole person, body and mind. Whether you use kitchen pharmacy all the time or just now and then, you will soon get to know the basic principles and will find that many of the treatments are largely based on common sense.

TOO MUCH YANG AND HEAT

The symptoms of too much yang are excessive heat in the body; redness in the whole face, not just the cheeks; a craving for coolness. There may be inflammation, dryness, red rashes on the skin, restlessness, a strong tendency towards anger, loudness, impatience and aggression. Sometimes there are 'bursting'-type symptoms like headaches; various types of high blood pressure, and also hyperactivity. The pulse is quite rapid and feels strong, and the tongue may be red. The urine is dark and copious.

Remedies for this condition are: mung beans, tofu and seaweeds; most vegetables, except onions, garlic, horseradish and leeks. Most fruits are recommended. If you are not vegetarian try to eat fish and poultry in moderation, and avoid red meats. Be very moderate in your intake of alcohol, coffee, hot spices, salt and fried foods. Mint, lemon grass, lemon verbena, rosehips and hibiscus are recommended, also

ROSE JAM (see page 77). If you need to take herbal tonics try those which are cooling like licium, plantain, borage and American ginseng. Avoid hot tonics and stimulants like guarana and common ginseng. Relaxation exercises would be helpful to counteract impulsiveness and anger; and you could try the following essential oils: geranium, grapefruit, lavender, lemon, rose and jasmine.

TOO LITTLE YANG (OR EMPTY-YANG) AND COLDNESS

In this condition, the person feels cold, with cold limbs and lower back, and a tendency to chills which are worse in winter. The complexion is pale, the sexual desire low, the pulse slow and weak, and the tongue pale. There is a feeling of general tiredness and the person gets fatigued easily. There is frequent pale urine.

Remedies are needed to warm the body and help to raise the yang. These are hot vegetables and spices such as fennel, garlic, ginger, cinnamon, cloves, horseradish, mustard, nutmeg, oregano, rosemary, sage, savory, thyme, chillies, leeks, and onions. Most vegetables can be eaten, preferably steamed or sautéed and slightly warmed with some of the spices mentioned above. In winter fruits can be eaten in moderation and particularly if baked; raw vegetables and salads can be eaten, but again in moderation. Too many oranges, bananas, pears, grapes and mangoes should be avoided, as should too much pineapple, dried fruit and sweet foods. Good herbal tonics are common ginseng, schizandra, solidago and astragalus; and helpful essential oils are ginger, rosemary, juniper and sage.

TOO LITTLE YIN OR EMPTY-YIN

The body needs a good level of moisture and coolness to counterbalance the processes of combustion and heat, and sometimes the equilibrium is disturbed. In the case of empty-yin the symptoms are sometimes confused with too much yang; in fact the problem is not too much yang but too little yin to balance it. Symptoms of empty-yin are: pale face with red dots on the cheeks, also known as 'malor flush'; very dry skin; tendency to dry coughs with an inflamed throat; hot palms and soles of feet, particularly at night. Some very important symptoms are night sweats, hot flushes and feverishness in the afternoon. There is a sense of listlessness and fatigue, and symptoms can get worse in very hot weather. The pulse is rapid but weak and the urine is scanty but frequent and dark. The tongue could be scarlet, cracked or peeled.

In some food cures, including some based on macrobiotics, this condition is often wrongly described as being too yin, because the person can look tired and depleted. If this condition is treated with a warming diet to raise the yang it can be made worse. What is needed is a diet containing foods which are not only cooling but which also have moistness in them, since moisture is a very yin agent. Alcohol, coffee, red meats, hot spices, fried food and hot tonics like guarana and common ginseng should be avoided.

Foods which are helpful include: salads (particularly in summer), raw and cooked vegetables and fruits; in particular, artichokes, pumpkin, dandelion, wild chicory (not the white English salad chicory), lettuce, seaweeds, melon, pawpaw, peaches; also millet, mung beans and tofu; rosehips, hibiscus, rose tea, and ROSE JAM (see page 77). Good herbal tonics are violet leaves or flowers, licium, rehmania; and of the essential oils, geranium, rose and vetivert.

STUCK CHI

Chi in Chinese means 'energy'. The Chinese considered the free flow of energy to be very important. If it did not flow, it resulted in a condition known as 'stuck chi', or stuck energy. Stuck chi very often affects the digestive system, which naturally has a downward flow of energy from the stomach, through the intestines. The energy in the digestive system can get stuck and go up instead of down, creating conditions such as bloating, hiccups and heartburn. The person often feels rather frustrated and nervous and may find that their digestive system seems to get blocked.

Symptoms of stuck chi are: bloating or distension, soreness (but not stabbing pain); the feeling of a lump, which is often gas; hiccups, belching and flatulence. Stuck chi is improved by exercise and movement, as well as by taking certain herbs, spices and other foods.

It is important with stuck chi not to eat stodgy and heavy meals which block the digestion and hamper the downward flow of chi. So you should go carefully on the following foods, eating them in moderation only: flour products, like bread, cakes, scones, biscuits and pasta (particularly white); potatoes and bananas. Too much sugar, including honey and dried fruits, can also slow the chi, and too many cold drinks can have a cramping and blocking effect on the digestion. On the other hand, hot spices raise the yang energy upwards and disturb the downward flow of energy, so the keyword for this condition is moderation, and the best advice is to chew all food well.

The balanced diet described on pages 31–8 is most appropriate, and recommended spices and teas are: fennel, bay leaf, caraway, cumin, coriander, mint, orange peel and tarragon. For the nervousness associated with this condition, camomile, aniseed and lemon verbena are helpful; and essential oils of mint, orange peel, grapefruit peel, mandarin peel, fennel and aniseed are all beneficial.

STAGNANT BLOOD

According to Chinese medicine, energy moves the blood. If this energy becomes stuck, as in stuck chi, the result may be a condition described as stagnant blood. This condition frequently affects women.

The symptoms of stagnant blood are broken capillaries, dark purple spots on the skin, purple varicose veins and stabbing pains. These pains are often experienced by women before a period or during the first day of menstruation, with dark clots in the blood. The liver is very often affected, too. In Chinese medicine the liver is considered to be largely responsible for the free flow of energy in the body. Both stuck chi and stagnant blood are often related to feelings of frustration and irritation; the energy which wants to express itself creatively and vibrantly is blocked and inhibited. There may also be suppression of other emotions.

Follow the same advice on diet and remedies as for stuck chi. Smoking hardens the arteries and so should be avoided if possible. The advice given under PREMENSTRUAL TENSION (page 228) and DYSMENORRHOEA or PAINFUL PERIODS (page 229) is appropriate for women suffering from stagnant blood. Read also the advice given under **The Heart and Circulatory System** on page 243. Massage the limbs often with combined essential oils of lavender and cypress (see page 45).

DAMPNESS

This condition is often experienced by people living in humid countries or damp surroundings (such as basements). Others who may be affected are those who do jobs such as cooking, where there is a great deal of vapour, or jobs where they have to keep their body in water for much of the time. The main symptom of dampness is a feeling of swelling, as if there is liquid underneath the skin. This may be in the abdomen, although it affects the joints particularly, and, according to Chinese medicine, is one of the main causes of RHEUMATISM (page 237). There may be a sense of dull pressure on the head, and lethargy. Dampness gives a feeling of heaviness and turbidity. An accumulation of dampness in the body can create conditions such as LEUCORRHOEA or EXCESSIVE VAGINAL DISCHARGE (page 230).

There are two types of dampness: cold dampness and hot dampness. Cold dampness is more frequent during the winter. There is often swelling with cramp-like pains, as in rheumatic pain. There may be a white coating on the tongue. If there are discharges, they are likely to be white, and the person feels chilly and cold.

In hot dampness or damp heat, there is more swelling, with redness and burning, and the discharges tend to be more yellow in colour. Hot dampness is more common in hot, humid countries, although it can also occur in cold countries as a result of eating too many fried and spicy foods. All forms of dampness are aggravated by eating fatty or oily food.

For both types of dampness, avoid pork in all its forms; sugar and sweetened foods; dairy produce, except for some yogurt and a little cottage cheese; fried and greasy food. If the problem is cold dampness, avoid cold, stodgy, moist foods, like pineapple, grapes, mangoes, bananas, white bread and pasta, particularly during cold weather. You can use some warming spices like cinnamon, cloves, ginger, thyme, oregano and savory. Drink ginger and cinnamon teas and add 5 or 6 drops of the essential oils of ginger and juniper to your bath. See also the advice given under COLD JOINT PROBLEMS (page 238).

When hot dampness is the problem, avoid pork, sugar, fried and fatty foods, dairy produce and alcohol. Follow the balanced diet described on pages 31–8, and include mint, rosehips, apples, quinces, wild berries, melon, lemon, lemon thyme, lemon grass, carrots, courgettes, cabbage, asparagus and pumpkin. See the advice given under HOT JOINT PROBLEMS (page 239).

MUCUS OR PHLEGM

This very common condition is seen as an advanced form of dampness, and also as a sign of digestive weakness, in as far as the digestive system is being overloaded with, or is unable to eliminate, fatty substances. The respiratory system can often be affected, creating a runny or blocked nose with mucus, phlegm or catarrh; or there can be mucus in the chest. Sometimes the mucus might be loose so that the person can bring it up, or it could be stuck, so that although there is a great deal of rattling in the chest, the person cannot expectorate. The mucus is sometimes in the stools as well, as is the case in ulcerative colitis or dysentery; or, as mentioned in the previous condition of dampness, the mucus can also show itself in discharges from the genital organs.

As with dampness, mucus can be either cold or hot. When the mucus is cold, it is white or transparent, and the person feels chilly. In hot mucus, the colour is yellow, green or brown and is accompanied by symptoms of heat in the body. In both cases of phlegm, particularly during the acute stage, it is very important to avoid dairy produce, except for a little yogurt (see ANTI-MUCUS DIET, page 39). In conditions of cold phlegm you should also avoid too many cold and moist foods like raw fruits. Follow a balanced diet (pages 31–8), adding ginger, clover, garlic, mustard, horseradish, leeks and onions, as they all warm and help to bring up the phlegm. Take care, though, not to overheat your system. In hot phlegm you must avoid the foods mentioned in the anti-mucus diet, and take both cooling foods and also the warming foods, as for cold phlegm, in moderation.

EMPTY OR WEAK BLOOD

Empty or weak blood resembles the condition known in the West as anaemia and the treatment is similar. The Chinese also aim to describe the energetic quality of the blood and its volume, or how much of it there is in the body. Certain types of anaemia, like pernicious anaemia, need medical supervision.

Symptoms of empty or weak blood are: pale face, lassitude, weak nails; brittle hair with split ends; hazy vision; dizziness and dry skin. In women, there could be scanty and pale periods.

Follow a balanced diet (pages 31–8), adding dried peaches, apricots, dates and figs; spinach, shiitake mushrooms, beetroot, dandelion, radicchio, watercress, parsley, beans and lentils, oatmeal, artichoke, wild berries and powdered yeast. If you are not vegetarian, include lamb liver, cockles and sardines. You might find drinking Guinness helpful, and the following herbal tonics are recommended: dang quai, cooked rehmania, nettle, and yellow dock.

Self-Diagnosis

Once you have ascertained whether you have one or more of these conditions, find the area of your body which seems to be most affected by it, and then look under the relevant heading in the chapter on 'Ailments' for further advice.

Alternatively, you can make a systematic self-diagnosis in the following way. Take a piece of paper and write down all your symptoms, beginning with your head and working right down your body. If you get headaches, note what they feel like; then look at the section on **Headaches and Migraine** (page 259) and read the diet advised for that condition. Do the same with your respiratory, digestive, urinary and other systems. You will often find that the advice given under one system will also apply to another system. This is because the same energy imbalance may be affecting several parts of the body: for instance, a hot type of headache might go along with a hot liver problem.

If, on the other hand, you find that you have two opposite conditions, such as a hot headache and a cold mucus condition in your lungs, both need to be treated. You can combine two different dishes in one meal, one for each condition. Or you can look after one condition in one meal and another in the next.

What Makes a Balanced Diet?

The foundation of all the treatments described in the following pages is a healthy, balanced diet, and we would like to clarify what we mean by this.

Scientific research is currently making rapid progress in the field of nutrition; many traditional approaches are being rediscovered, and there is much conflicting and confusing advice about what makes a healthy diet. For instance, some people recommend a diet of mainly raw vegetables, whilst others say that cooked vegetables and brown rice are best; some people advise a high-protein diet, others a low-protein one. Some people say butter is best; others, margarine, olive oil or other vegetable oils. Faced with all this conflicting advice, what sort of diet should one follow?

In this book we have done our best to avoid rigid dogmas and one-sided opinions in order to give you as balanced a view as possible. Remember that, having tried various approaches, you are the final judge and you have to make your own decisions, based on how your body feels and what works for you.

Traditional Chinese medicine can be a great help in making these decisions, because it makes us realise that different diets suit us best at different times, according to the state of our energies and the season of the year. Therefore it is not a question of one dogma against another, but rather a question of what we need at a certain time. Chinese medicine also gives us general guidance as to what proportions of different foods make up a basically healthy diet and we can adapt this accordingly. The percentages refer to the amount of space each item takes up on your plate.

A balanced diet might consist of:

30–40 per cent wholegrains such as oats, oat bran, millet, brown rice, buckwheat, wheat, barley and maize. (This includes potatoes and cooked plantain.)

30–40 per cent vegetables, more cooked ones in winter, and more raw ones in summer. Again, if you have a hot temperament, you might want to eat more raw vegetables; if a cold one, then more cooked. (This includes seaweeds, too.)

10–20 per cent proteins from vegetable sources, or animal if you are non-vegetarian. Pulses are a good form of protein; if you are a non-vegetarian, try to eat some vegetable protein regularly instead of animal.

10–20 per cent fruits and nuts, including dried fruits. Do not eat more dried fruits and nuts in a day than you can hold in your slightly clenched fist, as they can be rather heavy to digest. Again, follow the seasons and your own energy levels; you will need more fresh fruits during hot summer months and if you have a hot constitution. Dried fruits and nuts are warming if you have a cold constitution.

In general you should aim for a diet which is high in cereals and vegetables, and, thus, fibre; low in sugar and fat. You can still enjoy a wide range of delicious foods; and, if you are healthy, you can certainly have the occasional treat or binge. Such a diet is a joyful way of life; the food is easy to cook and a pleasure to eat. It's never too late to improve your eating habits and, in doing so, you will not only assist the healing of specific ailments but also greatly benefit your general health.

HOW MUCH WATER SHOULD YOU DRINK?

This really depends on individual temperament. To drink too much or too little fluid can unduly tax the digestive system. First of all, have mineral or filtered water. If you are filtering your water, make sure that you change the filter regularly, at least once a month, to avoid a harmful build-up of bacteria. It is important to ensure that the water you are drinking does not contain high levels of either sodium or calcium. Read the label on bottled mineral water, or, in the case of filtered tap water, ask your local Water Authority. The sodium content should not be above 25 mg per litre and the calcium not above 60 mg per litre.

Our liquid intake is also determined by how much table salt or sodium we eat; the more we use, the more we need to drink. Equally, when your diet is high in animal proteins, you need to drink more water in order to flush the toxins out. But if a diet is low in sodium and animal proteins and has a good proportion of vegetables and fruits, then natural thirst will be the best guide as to how much fluid is needed. Drinking beer, wine or coffee does not have the same cleansing effect as drinking water. On the contrary, these drinks intoxicate our system. Neither should fruit juices be our main source of liquid because although their sugar content is natural too much of it can also cause an imbalance in the system.

Try and drink at least one hour before or after meals; too much liquid with food bloats you up, slows digestion and hampers assimilation. Particularly if you are a rather cold person, or mainly vegetarian, or on a very low sodium diet, too much fluid will be of no service to you.

Do not have chilled drinks with meals; they should be at room temperature, or you could have a cup of a lukewarm tea such as green tea, mint, fennel, orange peel, lemon verbena, rosehip or cardamom. Try to limit yourself to one cup.

The Japanese macrobiotic diet hit the headlines several times in the past because some of its followers became severely ill on it. One of the major disadvantages of this diet is that a high level of sodium – in products such as miso, tamari, tekka, seaweeds and umeboshi plums – is combined with a minimal intake of liquid. If you decide to follow this diet, watch these points.

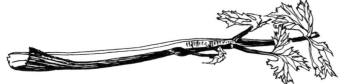

WHAT ABOUT ORGANICALLY PRODUCED FOOD?

When available and affordable, try to eat mainly organically produced food. Look for food in as natural a state as possible, without added colouring, emulsifiers, preservatives and other chemical additives. Your body will certainly benefit.

WHAT ABOUT MEAT AND FISH?

We would like to encourage people to heal themselves with non-animal food. However, some people are suspicious of vegetarianism because they think such a diet will not contain sufficient nutrients. In some cases they might be right. For instance, vegetarians who adopt a diet based on refined cereals and white sugar will certainly lack some minerals and vitamins. On the other hand, if one follows a vegetarian or semi-vegetarian diet which is balanced, as advised in this book, then there is no risk of any such deficiency. On the contrary, there are many benefits, as shown by many scientific studies on vegetarian groups such as the Seventh Day Adventists.

For those who prefer to follow a non-vegetarian diet we describe the properties of meat, poultry and fish at the end of the 'Remedies' chapter, on pages 203–6.

WHICH FAT IS BEST FOR HEALTH?

The question of which fat is the healthiest to use is still a controversial one. However, nutritionists and researchers generally agree that we need to reduce our intake of fat, and, in particular, of saturated fat. Saturated fat is solid at room temperature and is found in meat, lard, butter, cheese, cream, eggs and some vegetable fats (specifically, palm oil and coconut oil). It is also found in margarines which do not state that they are high in polyunsaturates and have not been hydrogenated.

In recent years many experts have advised the use of polyunsaturated fats (fats which are liquid at room temperature, including corn oil, sunflower oil, grapeseed oil and soya oil), because they help to lower cholesterol levels in the blood. In doing so, however, they remove from the blood not only the low-density lipoproteins (LDLs) which deposit cholesterol on the arteries, but also the high-density lipoproteins (HDLs) which help the body to get rid of it.

Research has shown that when polyunsaturated oils become rancid or are heated (as happens in the production of most margarines) a chemical reaction takes place in which substances called free radicals are produced. Free radicals are molecules which can have a negative effect on the body, causing premature aging, atherosclerosis and other health disorders.

Bearing these considerations in mind, some experts now believe that it is best to use a monosaturated oil, such as olive oil, which does not produce free radicals, and which helps the body to get rid of LDLs whilst still keeping HDLs. Others still consider that the advantages of poly-unsaturated oils outweigh the disadvantages. And there are those who still consider butter to be the best choice.

The recipes in this book specify olive oil. However, the decision is obviously yours. You may prefer to use one of the polyunsaturated seed oils for cooking and keep olive oil for salad dressings and other cold dishes.

Amidst all the confusion, a number of pointers to healthy eating emerge:

- Cut down on your total fat intake as much as possible.
- If you use margarine, make sure that it is a polyunsaturated type produced at low temperatures and is unhydrogenated; ask at your local healthfood shop.
- When you buy polyunsaturated oils, choose cold-pressed ones, and if you are cooking with them – for instance, stir-frying or sautéeing at the beginning of a recipe – use the minimum of oil and do not let it get very hot.
- Keep oils well stoppered in a dark, cool place; once they have been opened, it is best to keep them in the fridge.
- Fry food as little as possible and do not re-use oil or fat.
- Steam, bake and grill foods whenever you can; delicious virgin olive oil, or a mixture of olive oil and a cold-pressed polyunsaturated oil, plus other flavourings such as lemon juice and herbs, can be added after cooking.
- Virgin olive oil or cold-pressed polyunsaturated oils can be used in salad dressings.
- Remember that nuts and seeds contain valuable polyunsaturated oils. You can eat a few each day, but make sure they are really fresh, with no sign of rancidity. To ensure this, it is best to buy nuts in their shells if possible. Seeds, shelled nuts and wheatgerm are best stored in the fridge or freezer.

SHOULD TEA AND COFFEE BE RESTRICTED?

It's advisable to cut down on tea and coffee. Try replacing them with herb teas such as rosehip, hibiscus, mint, fennel, lemon verbena, lemon or orange peel; or with coffee substitutes made from roasted cereals, chicory or dandelion. Decaffeinated coffee is not necessarily a good choice because the residues of the chemical solvents used to remove the caffeine may have a worse effect than the caffeine itself. However, healthfood shops sell organic coffee which has been decaffeinated through carbon filters.

WHAT ABOUT SUGAR AND OTHER SWEETENERS?

In our opinion, white sugar is one of the worst foods for health. Although the body needs sugar for energy, it can get plenty from vegetables, fruit and grains. Sugar in these forms is absorbed slowly because, firstly, their natural fibre means that these foods have to be chewed, thus taking time to reach the digestive tract; and secondly, once there, the sugar can be gently extracted from the fibre without straining the pancreas.

In contrast, when we eat refined sugar, it hits the digestive system fast, with no fibre to slow things up, and the pancreas has to take emergency action. The effect of white sugar on the pancreas has been likened to a sleeping person having a bucket of ice-cold water tipped over them. The initial burst of energy is followed by a 'low', so that we feel the urge to eat more sugar for another boost, and so the vicious circle continues. In the process, teeth are harmed, digestion impaired and absorption of many nutrients impeded.

White sugar can be replaced by raw Barbados sugar – the kind which looks really sticky, dark and treacly and which contains some vitamins and minerals; by fresh and dried fruits; apple juice concentrate, maple syrup, date syrup and honey. Even these should, however, be taken in moderation, since too much sugar of any kind can strain the pancreas. They are of course inadvisable if a person is hypoglycaemic.

Honey is neutral and moist. It lubricates the intestines and lungs, relieving symptoms such as constipation, dry coughs and sore throats; it also soothes inflammation, especially in the digestive and respiratory organs. Honey gives energy whilst at the same time soothing nervous tension, so it is helpful for people who are tired and stressed. Honey is not advised for people who are lethargic or overweight, or who have conditions such as hypoglycaemia and diabetes.

Other products made by bees – royal jelly, pollen and propolis – can also be useful. Royal jelly is a highly nourishing food which increases resistance to disease, builds up yin energy and helps us put on weight. Some researchers have recently claimed that they cannot find any substances in royal jelly to substantiate claims made for it; however, we feel that, as in the case of vitamin C and scurvy, its properties may in time be explained.

Pollen contains many nutrients and increases vigour and resistance to illness; being warmer in nature than royal jelly, it is particularly helpful in building up yang energy. Propolis has a very powerful natural antibiotic action which is helpful for various infections.

Molasses, the thick black syrup extracted during the refining of cane sugar, contains large amounts of minerals such as iron and calcium. It is therefore a good blood tonic and a useful supplement if taken in moderation – 1–2 teaspoons a day – when necessary. It can be used to give extra nourishment and energy during times of unusual physical and mental activity. Molasses lubricates the intestines and lungs, helping constipation, dry coughs and sore throats. In India it is also considered to be a good liver tonic, especially during recovery from jaundice or hepatitis. It should not be taken when there is diabetes, hypoglycaemia and obesity.

CUTTING DOWN ON SALT

Research has linked high salt intake with raised blood pressure, strokes and heart attacks. Cutting down on salt where possible certainly makes sense. The diet recommended in this book automatically reduces salt because it replaces canned and convenience foods with wholegrains, fruits and vegetables, and is low on cheese. Using an unsalted butter or margarine (available from healthfood shops) and low-salt vegetable stock cubes can also help. Try cooking rice and grains, and steaming vegetables, without salt, then adding GOMASIO, a mixture of roasted ground sesame seeds and salt (see page 172), at the table. We also recommend miso, a nutritious savoury paste made from soya beans, and the natural soy sauces, tamari and shoyu. These ingredients are all high in salt, as are seaweeds, and need to be used with care. A potassium-based salt substitute such as Biosalt can be a useful alternative to ordinary salt.

ARE VITAMIN AND MINERAL SUPPLEMENTS NECESSARY?

Vitamin and mineral supplements can be helpful during times of stress, poor nutrition, illness, convalescence and rapid growth. Take natural vitamins, from healthfood shops, rather than synthesised ones. Remember that if you take high doses of a single vitamin or mineral over a prolonged period it can deplete the body of other nutrients. As in so many dietary matters, moderation is the key.

Fish oil supplements have received some publicity because of studies showing that there is a low incidence of heart disease amongst Eskimos, who consume them in large quantities. However, research has also revealed that Eskimos are extremely prone to other diseases, including strokes. The issue is therefore unclear and we do not advise taking high dosages of these oils.

Diets for Specific Purposes

ANTI-INFLAMMATION DIET

This diet is useful whenever there is acute inflammation in the body. The aim is to nourish the body without putting any extra stress on it, and to help speed up the healing process. It is quite a restricted diet but is not generally followed for very long periods. On this diet, you eat only the following foods: very well-cooked wholegrains, especially brown rice, barley and millet; steamed courgettes, pumpkin, carrot, cabbage and fennel bulb (these can be puréed if you like, and can be served with a very small amount of extra virgin olive oil as a flavouring). The vegetables can be eaten together, or, for the sake of variety, you can just have one type, along with brown rice, millet or maize, for each main meal. With the vegetables and grains you can have a small amount of tofu, or steamed white fish if you eat this; these should not make up more than 10–15 per cent of your plate. The only permissible fruits are the occasional baked apple, pear or quince; and the only teas are lemon verbena, mint and the occasional cup of camomile.

YEAST-FREE DIET

On this diet you need to stop eating yeast and all products containing it, such as yeast extract; all wheat products, especially bread and pasta; dairy products, with the exception of a little very low-fat yogurt; mushrooms; both white and brown sugar, honey, and all products containing these; tomatoes; all fruits except the occasional apple; alcohol; coffee; all fermented products, including vinegar, pickles and miso. This means that your diet will essentially consist of brown rice and other grains (except for wheat) and a wide range of herbs, vegetables, pulses and tofu, spices and herb teas.

ANTI-MUCUS DIET

This diet cuts out rich dairy produce, especially fatty cheese and milk (at most, you could have a little very low-fat yogurt and cottage cheese perhaps once a week); refined cereals, especially bread and pasta; meat such as pork; and fried and fatty foods. All these foods encourage the body to produce mucus which then accumulates in the respiratory system, exacerbating many of its problems. Although this may seem a very restricted diet, there is still a wide range of fruits, vegetables, grains, pulses, nuts, sugarless cakes, and, for non-vegetarians, fish and chicken from which to make delicious meals.

ANTI-CHOLESTEROL DIET

The basic balanced diet described on page 32 will go a long way towards preventing heart disease and improving the health of your heart. In addition to those recommendations, in order to reduce cholesterol your diet should exclude all fatty cheeses, cream and ice-cream; hydrogenated fat, which includes most margarines; fried food and pork. You need to cut down on milk and butter; red meat, including minced meat and dishes made from this, such as hamburgers; alcohol, coffee and salt; refined grains such as white bread and flour; sugar and foods which contain it. Eggs can be eaten in moderation: that is, one or two a week.

If you like margarine, make sure that it is not hydrogenated because this process makes the oils in it turn saturated. Most healthfood shops now have unhydrogenated margarines, with the added bonus that they do not contain salt or artificial colourings and preservatives. You can use a little oil in your cooking, but keep to olive oil or seed oils like maize/corn or sunflower. In salads use mainly extra virgin olive oil, lemon juice and a little natural wine or cider vinegar; this is a very good combination to reduce cholesterol.

Most wholegrains are good but maize, rye and buckwheat have a particularly helpful action on the circulatory system. Oatflakes and oatmeal, perhaps made into PORRIDGE (see page 160), and sprinkled with oat bran and oatgerm, are also recommended for cholesterol.

Bear in mind, too, that the following foods are good for helping to reduce cholesterol and fatty deposits, so include them as often as possible (providing, of course, that they are not inadvisable for any other conditions you may have): grapefruit, melon, apples, pawpaw, bilberries, lemon, lime, mandarins, oranges; most salads and vegetables, particularly dandelion, cabbage, artichoke, garlic, onions, leeks, pulses, celery and seaweeds; also fresh lime or lemon juice, which you can take in hot or cold water, or in your tea.

FASTING

Fasting can sometimes be helpful, to cleanse the body and give the digestive system a rest. It is important both to go into a fast, and to come out of it, gently. So, for two or three days before your fast, eat simply and lightly, perhaps in a similar way to that described for the ANTI-INFLAMMA-TION DIET (page 38). For the actual fast, try to choose two or three days when you can take life in a reasonably relaxed way: a quiet weekend is ideal. Just drink filtered or mineral water (see page 32), fruit juice, or a CLEAR VEGETABLE BROTH (see page 86). After your fast, slowly introduce solid food, perhaps again following the ANTI-INFLAMMATION DIET for a day or two, then gradually adding other foods.

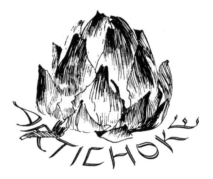

3

The Remedies and How to Use Them –
The Materia Medica

Here you will find descriptions of around 120 remedies, their properties and how to use them both to maintain health, to treat common ailments and improve chronic ones. The Materia Medica complements the 'Ailments' chapter, which gives more detailed and specific guidance on treating individual conditions.

Flowers, Herbs and Spices

Amongst the flowers, herbs and spices are some of nature's most potent healers, a number of which have been used since prehistoric times. The ones described here are those we have found most useful. With the exception of the flowers and rosehips, for which you may need to go to a shop specialising in herbs, all the herbs and spices mentioned are the ordinary kind which are used in cooking and are widely available, often both dried and fresh, at shops and supermarkets. You can also use ready-made herb teas if these contain the particular ingredient or blend you need. Sometimes we refer to the tincture of a herb or spice, and in many cases to the essential oil. We begin this section with instructions on making decoctions, infusions, tinctures, compresses, poultices, massage oils and ointments, together with practical points on the general use of these products. The descriptions of the individual herbs and spices follow, arranged in alphabetical order.

BUYING, STORING AND USING HERBS AND SPICES

Fresh herbs, full of fragrance and flavour, are a joy to use when you can get them. However, they are not always available and in most cases dried herbs will do just as well. Unless we specifically refer to fresh herbs, the quantities given in the descriptions and recipes are for dried herbs. If you are using fresh herbs you will need approximately twice the amount. Even when they have been dried, herbs and spices are best used as soon as possible, so buy them from a shop which has a quick turnover and use them up quickly. Keep them well-stoppered in jars, preferably away from the light to ensure freshness.

Spices always have more flavour and potency if you buy them whole, and grind or crush them as you need them. They can be crushed with a wooden spoon on a board, but a pestle and mortar, or a small electric coffee grinder, kept for the purpose, make the job easier. If you are buying a pestle and mortar, we recommend a ceramic one, rather than one made of wood, because wood can take on the flavour of particular spices and is difficult to clean.

Most herbs and spices can be used to make teas and also to flavour all sorts of foods, ranging from soups and salads to main courses, sweet dishes, breads, cakes and biscuits; they can be forked into cooked rice or other grains, mixed with pasta or mashed potato, sprinkled over steamed or sautéed vegetables or baked potatoes, eaten on toast or in sandwiches, added to stewed, baked, fresh or dried fruits. Some of them can be chewed or eaten just as they are.

Alternatively, they can be made into gargles, hair rinses, compresses or poultices, or added to a bath or foot-bath; detailed instructions, where these apply, are given under the individual herb, spice or flower. Herbs are sometimes used, too, in the form of a decoction, a solution produced by boiling the herbs in water, which is often stronger than a tea or infusion. They can be taken as a tincture, a liquid produced by steeping herbs in a mixture of alcohol and water, a particularly convenient way of taking herbal medicine.

Making an Infusion or Tea: An infusion or tea should be made with water which has just boiled. It is often easiest to make tea in the cup, with a pinch to a teaspoonful of the required herb or spice, depending on its potency. If you are using a teapot, increase the amount accordingly; and with fresh herbs use double the amount and either chop or snip them, or use the leaves or sprigs whole, crushing them a little with a spoon to release their fragrance and oils. You can use one variety or a mixture. Pour the water over the herbs or spices; let the tea infuse for 5–10 minutes, then strain it if you like. Lemon and honey can be added to taste unless these are inadvisable for your particular condition. Teas can also be taken cold, which is refreshing in hot weather and useful if you have a condition which needs cooling.

It is usually recommended that you should not take one type of medicinal tea every day for more than 3 weeks at a time. After that, stop for a week or 10 days. You can repeat this course a further 3 times before stopping. This applies to teas such as aniseed, rosemary, thyme and oregano, not to common, widely available herbal teas such as mint and rosehip, which you can drink freely. With warming teas, such as ginger, notice how you are feeling, and stop taking them, or reduce the frequency, if you experience any slight burning sensation in throat and stomach, or symptoms of overheating, such as red face and eyes.

Making a Decoction: To make a decoction, put 15 g/½ oz herbs into a saucepan with 600 ml/1 pint cold water. Bring to the boil and simmer for the required amount of time. This is usually 15 minutes, although it can vary according to the type of herb you are using. Allow it to cool, covered.

Tinctures: Tinctures can be bought from healthfood shops and herbalists. When they are professionally produced they are made by steeping the plants in a mixture of alcohol and water, the exact proportions varying from plant to plant, to produce a tincture which is approximately 20 per cent alcohol. However, you can make a tincture at home by putting 225 g/8 oz chopped fresh herbs or half that amount of dried herbs into a jar with 300 ml/½ pint (75 per cent proof) Polish vodka and 250 ml/8 fl oz water. Cover tightly and keep in a warm place for 2 weeks, shaking the jar twice a day, then strain through muslin and keep well-stoppered in a dark glass bottle.

The usual dose is 25–30 drops of a tincture in half a glass of water 2–3 times a day. When a higher concentration is required, a teaspoonful can be taken in water twice a day, but this is best taken under supervision. When a strong cleansing action is required, for a condition such as a tumour, the prescription is often to put 1–2 tablespoons tincture into 1 litre/1¾ pints water and to sip this throughout the day.

For instructions on treating children with tinctures, see page 12.

Making a Compress: A compress is a pad of soft material wrung out in water or a herbal mixture and applied to the body. To make a compress, soak a piece of clean cloth or cottonwool in a decoction or infusion of the appropriate herb or mixture of herbs, then put the cloth or cottonwool on the affected part. If you want a hot compress, sometimes called a fomentation, the herbal mixture should be hot, and you can keep the compress warm by putting a hot water bottle on top of it. For a cooling action, use cold liquid. Keep renewing the compress as necessary.

Making a Poultice: A poultice, which may sometimes also be called a fomentation, is a soft moist mixture, generally hot, which is applied to the skin. To make a poultice, mix the herbs or powdered spices to a thick paste with water, spread on a piece of gauze or cheesecloth and apply with the cloth next to the skin. Cover with another piece of fabric or an old towel.

BUYING, STORING AND USING ESSENTIAL OILS

Essential oils are non-greasy, highly concentrated, aromatic extracts from plants with, in our experience, and that of many who have tried them, powerful healing properties.

It is very important to use good-quality oils. These will always be in dark bottles, never in clear glass, which allows the oil to deteriorate in the light, nor in plastic, which reacts detrimentally with the oils. The label will tell you the name of the oil and also the Latin name of the plant from which it has been extracted.

The price of different oils varies vastly, according to the rarity of the plant from which they have been extracted, and the amount of oil the plant contains, so pure essential oils should vary in price within a range if they are genuine. Avoid any oils labelled 'aromatherapy oil', which will probably have been diluted; or 'perfume oil', which is most likely to be synthetic; and oils which have had anything added to or taken away from them. Oils extracted from organically grown plants are the best, when you can get them. Good-quality essential oils can be bought from some herbalists and healthfood shops, or you can get them by post (see page 289). A reputable shop will usually make up a small quantity of the most expensive oils, such as rose, jasmine, camomile and orange flower (neroli), mixed with a base oil, say 10 drops of essential oil in 1 teaspoon base oil, so that you can try them at a more reasonable price.

Essential oils should be kept tightly stoppered in a cool, dark place, away from direct sunlight. They should also be kept away from vibrations and loud noises as these can upset their delicate balance. With care, they will keep for several years.

These oils can be added to baths or foot-baths; sprinkled on to a handkerchief or pillow and sniffed; added to oil and used for massage; or, sometimes, applied straight to wounds, added to hair or face rinses or lotions or gargles. They can also be burnt, or evaporated, either diluted in water or neat (which we think is best) on a special burner over a nightlight. Because of their highly volatile nature, you should only add essential oils just before you want to use them.

As with herbal teas, it's best not to continue using one particular type of oil for longer than about 14 days, or 3 weeks at the most; have a break, or try a different oil for a week or so. If you dislike the smell of an essential oil, do not use it. There is probably another which has a similar action which you can use instead.

Using Essential Oils in Baths and Foot-baths: Put 5–6 drops of essential oil into the bath just before you get in. Be careful about adding oils to a child's bath; in this case, use 1 drop in a baby bath, 2–3 drops in a normal bath used by a toddler and up to 4 drops for an older child. The essential oil should be diluted in 1 tablespoon oil, cream or milk before you add it to the bath. This is to avoid any risk of it getting on to the child's skin or into their eyes in too high a concentration. For a foot-bath, use 2–3 drops of essential oil.

Making a Massage Oil: This is one of the most convenient, soothing and effective ways of using essential oils. The essential oil has to be added to a vegetable oil, such as almond, sunflower or grapeseed oil; this is known as the 'base' or 'carrier' oil. Mix 4–5 drops of the essential oil in a saucer of base oil and gently rub some of this into the affected area. The exact quantities we recommend are 30 drops of essential oil to 100 ml/ 3½ fl oz base oil. This can be divided between different oils, but should not exceed 30 drops in all. For a smaller amount, use 1–2 drops of essential oil to 1 teaspoon almond or sunflower oil.

For instructions on making a massage oil for children, see page 12.

Double-Diluting an Essential Oil: A few of the essential oils, namely oregano, savory, thyme, cinnamon and cloves, are extremely hot, so these should be doubly diluted. To do this, first add 5 drops of the essential oil to 1 tablespoon almond, sunflower or grapeseed oil and mix well, then add this to 85 ml/3 fl oz massage oil.

Making an Ointment: An ointment can easily be made by mixing the required essential oils into a pure vegetable face cream which you can get from a healthfood shop. Choose a natural one without perfume or other additives. To a 65 g/2½ oz jar of cream, add 10 drops of essential oil or oils and mix gently.

ANISE (ANISEED) *Pimpinella anisum*

Neutral to slightly warming, digestive, calming, anti-spasmodic

Anise, or aniseed, is a small oval seed with a sweet, lingering liquorice-like flavour. Like many spices, it has been used since ancient times; it is mentioned frequently in Egyptian texts, the Vedas, the Bible and other ancient writings. Dioscorides, Pliny and Pythagoras praised its ability to 'perfume the breath and ease digestion'.

Aniseed has a calming action on the nervous system and, thus, on the digestive and respiratory systems which are so much affected by it. All forms of INDIGESTION are helped by aniseed, but especially those due to tension. It helps abdominal spasms, nausea, vomiting, hiccups and belching; it is also very suitable for COLIC in babies and young children. Aniseed can help INSOMNIA if it is due to digestive problems. It also has a mildly calming action on the lungs which is particularly useful for conditions such as ASTHMA or COUGHS.

Note: It is safe to use aniseed in moderation, or occasionally, for a few weeks at a time. By moderation we mean taking aniseed tea once a day for 3 weeks, then stopping for a week or 10 days, and repeating this course a further 3 times before stopping. If aniseed is used more frequently than this, it can over-sedate and excessively slow the metabolism.

Preparing and Using: Aniseed can be bought both whole and ground; the whole seeds are best and are quite soft so do not need grinding before use. For aniseed tea, infuse ¼–½ teaspoon aniseed in a cupful of boiling water for 5 minutes, then strain. A cupful of this tea can be taken once a day. In the case of a baby or toddler, give 1 teaspoon tea every 3–4 hours, until they improve.

The flavour of aniseed goes well with many vegetables, particularly carrots, cabbage, beetroot, courgettes, pumpkin, cucumber and pulses; add it to stir-fries or toss the cooked vegetables in melted butter or margarine and a sprinkling of aniseed. It's also good with fruits; try adding a pinch to baked or stewed plums, prunes, apples and pears (see the recipe for HONEYED PEARS WITH ANISEED on page 196). Sprinkle aniseed on home-made pastries, cakes or breads before baking; add to sweet or savoury biscuits or simply put on top of buttered biscuits or bread.

The essential oil of aniseed can be used externally. Mix 4–5 drops of the essential oil in a saucer of almond or sunflower oil and gently rub some of this into the abdomen, to ease pain and aid digestion.

BASIL *Ocymum basilicum*

Neutral, beneficial for the nerves

An annual plant native to India, basil has tender, aromatic leaves which have a flavour slightly reminiscent of cloves when fresh; of curry when dried.

Basil affects the nervous system, the head and brain, the digestive system and the lungs. As research by the French doctors, Cadeac and Meunier has shown, basil first stimulates the brain and nervous system, then calms them – an action similar to that of marjoram (see page 68). Like marjoram, mint, rosemary and orange leaves, basil is also reputed to sharpen the memory and may be helpful during times of mental effort, as when preparing for an examination.

Basil (again, like mint and marjoram) is reputed to relieve HEADACHES due to COLDS, INDIGESTION or NERVOUS TENSION. It will help expel a head cold or fever, and will ease abdominal cramps and swelling caused by indigestion and flatulence.

In the Mediterranean countries people believe that eating basil with the evening meal promotes sound sleep; and drinking basil tea first thing in the morning brings alertness.

Note: Basil tends to encourage menstruation so during pregnancy it should not be used in the form of the essential oil nor taken as a tea, although it can still be used as a flavouring in foods.

Preparing and Using: Make basil tea using ¼–½ teaspoon dried basil, or a good sprig of fresh basil, lightly crushed; flavour to taste with honey and lemon if you like.

Basil makes a deliciously refreshing ingredient in summer salads, especially those which contain tomato; try tomato, basil and avocado. It's also good in tomato sandwiches, or snipped over soups, pasta and freshly cooked vegetables. It goes particularly well with carrots, cabbage, courgettes, cucumber, lettuce, onions, potatoes, green beans, and, of course, tomatoes. Dried basil is good with lentils and pulses.

Add the essential oil to a massage oil and rub this on to the limbs to strengthen tense or flaccid muscles.

BAY LEAF *Laurus nobilis*

Warming, tonic, anti-spasmodic, diuretic, dry

The oval, leathery leaf of an evergreen tree, bay has a warm, vaguely resinous flavour, and a particularly helpful effect on the digestive system. Like fennel, thyme, mint and oregano, it helps break up and eliminate fats and, in addition, its diuretic action assists in the elimination of water and eases bloating. For these reasons, bay can be helpful for WEIGHT LOSS.

COLD RHEUMATISM – when the joints swell and feel worse in cold weather, with cramp-like pain – responds well to bay. For this, the essential oil can be used as a massage or 5 drops can be added to the bath.

Bay has a secondary expectorant action, helping to get rid of mucus and relieving COLDS and BRONCHITIS. It is a mild tonic and has a slightly euphoric quality, lifting the spirits. This may have been why the ancient Romans and Greeks believed that bay could bring happiness, and stimulate clairvoyance and artistic inspiration. Bay was worn by generals after victory as well as by poets and artists.

Note: Bay leaf tends to encourage menstruation so during pregnancy it should not be used in the form of the essential oil nor taken as a tea, although it can still be used as a flavouring in foods.

Preparing and Using: The leaves can be used either dried or fresh; the flavour is more intense when using dried leaves. Tear the leaves before using them, to help release the flavour and properties and add the leaf at the beginning of cooking.

One leaf of bay in a cupful of freshly boiled water is enough to make a pleasant, aromatic tea.

A leaf can also be added to any soup, casserole or vegetable dish; when cooking pulses or braising courgettes, pumpkin, marrow or cucumber in butter or olive oil. It can also be used to flavour milk for making sweet or savoury sauces and puddings or it can be added to a rice pudding before baking.

CAMOMILE (CHAMOMILE) *Matricaria recutita; Matricaria chamomilla*

Neutral, digestive, beneficial for the nerves

Camomile is a small plant of which the dried, golden-centred, white flowers are used; the fragrance and flavour are reminiscent of rather spicy farmyard hay.

The flowers have a strong action on the nervous system, reducing STRESS, calming TENSION and promoting peaceful sleep. They can help HEADACHES brought about by stress, over-concentration and NERVOUS INDIGESTION; indeed, camomile is one of the best teas for nervous indigestion, which causes stagnation and inflammation in the abdomen. Camomile is therefore useful for STOMACH CRAMPS, COLITIS, ULCERS, GASTRITIS, DIVERTICULITIS and similar conditions.

Any pain is made more bearable by taking camomile because of its mild analgesic action. This is especially true if the pain is of neuralgic origin, or along the nerves. Camomile slows a mild rapid heartbeat caused by tension and fear.

Note: Like all herbs and spices which have a calming effect on the system, if camomile is taken in excess it can cause lethargy and debilitation.

Preparing and Using: Camomile flowers are available from herbalists. If you cannot buy them, camomile tea is easy to get, either loose or made up into teabags.

On its own, or with orange flowers, camomile tea is relaxing and helps INSOMNIA when taken last thing at night; mixed with other digestive and calming herbs, such as aniseed, mint or orange peel, it is good after a meal.

The essential oil can be added to the bath, massaged over the abdomen, or all over the body. It can be applied to inflamed and sore areas, to soothe them. For this purpose camomile is best combined with essential oil of lavender, then mixed with a base oil in the usual way.

CARAWAY SEEDS, CUMIN SEEDS *Carum carvi, Cuminum cyminum*

Warm, digestive, anti-spasmodic

Both caraway and cumin seeds are long, thin and dark brown, cumin seeds being slightly paler than caraway. Caraway tastes sweet and spicy, rather like a mixture of pepper and liquorice; cumin is heavier, more pungent and slightly bitter. Both have a similar action to coriander seeds and fennel. They are generally tonic, but their main effect is on the

49

digestive system, where they help INDIGESTION by moving the energy down, easing hiccups, belching, swelling and flatulence due to putrefaction in the abdomen. These seeds stimulate the intestinal walls, helping spasms caused by flatulence and they also have a mild action against INTESTINAL PARASITES.

Note: It is not advisable to take caraway seeds or cumin seeds in the form of teas or essential oils during pregnancy or if suffering from prolonged or heavy periods since these seeds encourage menstruation. However, they can still be used as a flavouring in foods.

Preparing and Using: Caraway seeds are sold whole. Cumin may be either whole or ground; the whole seeds have a better flavour.

For caraway or cumin tea, use ½ teaspoon seeds to a cupful of boiling water.

Caraway and cumin seeds complement pulses and root vegetables particularly well, and caraway seeds are good with cabbage. Both can be sprinkled on top of breads and biscuits. And seed cake, a plain sponge with caraway seed added, was very popular in Victorian and Edwardian times.

For a soothing massage, mix the essential oil with almond or sunflower oil and rub into the abdomen.

SAVOURY CARAWAY AND RYE BISCUITS

Makes about 12.

> *100 g/4 oz rye flour*
> *a pinch of salt*
> *50 g/ 2 oz butter*
> *½ teaspoon caraway seeds*

Set the oven to 200°C/400°F/Gas Mark 6. Put the rye flour in a bowl with the salt, then rub in the butter until the mixture resembles breadcrumbs. Add the caraway seeds and then 4 teaspoons cold water, and mix to a dough. Turn out on to a board which has been sprinkled with rye flour and knead lightly. Roll out as thinly as you can and cut into round biscuits. Put on to a baking sheet, prick the biscuits lightly with a fork, then bake for 7–10 minutes, or until lightly browned. Allow the biscuits to cool on the baking sheet until they are firm enough to handle, then transfer them to a wire rack to finish cooling.

CARDAMOM SEEDS *Elettaria cardamomum*

Wind-expelling, aromatic

These small, dark brown seeds are contained within a ridged oval pod. They are highly aromatic, like a blend of eucalyptus, camphor and lemon; and they have one of the most pleasant aromas, cheering the heart, freshening the breath and speeding digestion.

Cardamom mixes well with other digestive aromatics, such as mint, fennel and aniseed, all of which move the energy down the abdomen. Cardamom is highly recommended for chronic INDIGESTION with bloating, belching, flatulence and hiccups. It relieves pressure in the chest and heart caused by a swollen stomach pressing on the diaphragm. Its mildly tonic properties are also helpful for weakness caused by STRESS and tense digestion.

Preparing and Using: It is best to buy whole cardamom; when removed from the pod or ground, the seeds quickly lose their flavour and fragrance.

Cardamom sweetens bad breath, especially if this is caused by poor digestion; chew a cardamom pod 2–3 times a day.

To make a delicious tea, infuse 2–3 pods in a cup of boiled water for 10 minutes. Alternatively, add cardamom pods to a normal pot of tea to make an aromatic brew.

The pods can be slightly crushed and sautéed with vegetables or added to rice or lentils before cooking, 3–4 to a cupful. Cardamom can also be infused in liquid to flavour ice-cream, sorbets and custards, or the seeds can be removed from the pods and added to cakes and biscuits.

Rub the diluted essential oil over the abdomen to stimulate the digestion.

CHILLI *Capsicum minimum*

Hot, stimulant, circulatory, mucus-expelling

Chillies are a pod-like variety of capsicum, hot and fiery to eat. They are hollow, containing white seeds, and may be red or green.

Like ginger, cloves and garlic, chillies have an antiseptic, warming and expectorant action on the respiratory system, promptly getting rid of mucus. As they bring on a sweat, they can be helpful in the first, 'shivery' stages of a COLD or FLU. The ability of chillies, like ginger, to

51

increase the circulation means that they are helpful for people with cold limbs and COLD RHEUMATISM.

Chillies are a stimulant, increasing vitality and digestive ability (and helping to ease CONSTIPATION) in cold, yin, lethargic people.

Note: Chillies should not be used by people with excess heat and inflammation in their system.

Preparing and Using: Chillies can be bought whole and fresh or whole and dried. They can also be dried and powdered, in the form of chilli powder and cayenne pepper, which are hot, and paprika pepper, which varies in heat but is generally milder. If you are using whole chillies, either fresh or dried, the seeds should first be removed. Be careful not to touch your face or eyes when preparing chillies and always wash your hands afterwards, to avoid irritation.

One chilli added to a recipe serving 2–4 people is usually hot enough for most people's taste, or, if you are using chilli powder or cayenne pepper, you could start with a pinch. Paprika can be used more generously. Chilli is excellent in bean and lentil dishes, particularly RED BEAN CHILLI (page 148) and LENTIL DAL (page 144). It's also good in spicy vegetable mixtures, and you can add it to CREAMY AVOCADO DIP (page 179) to make the Mexican dish guacamole.

CINNAMON *Cinnamomum*

Warming, tonic, expels colds, raises the yang, warms the digestive tract

Cinnamon is the dried inner bark from a small tree belonging to the laurel family. It has a warm, aromatic, slightly sweet flavour and is an ancient spice, used in many countries and mentioned in Chinese, Indian, Egyptian and Greek texts written hundreds of years before Christ. It is often referred to in the Old Testament, as in Exodus XXX, 23, where Moses is ordered to get some cinnamon for the anointing ceremony.

Laboratory tests both in China and France have shown that a decoction of cinnamon has an inhibiting effect on many organisms, including flu viruses and even salmonella typhi, which causes TYPHOID. This quality, together with its action in encouraging sweating, makes cinnamon valuable for COLDS AND FLU where there is a tendency towards chilliness and shivering.

As it warms the stomach and speeds up the digestive metabolism, cinnamon helps a SLOW DIGESTION with a cold abdomen. Flatulence, NAUSEA and DIARRHOEA are also helped by cinnamon, especially if these occur as a result of taking cold food.

Cinnamon is useful if you have weak yang energy and are often tired and cold; it relieves muscle pains due to cold weather or tiredness; and, like ginger and cloves, it is helpful for COLD RHEUMATISM where there is a cramping pain, and swelling which is worse in cold and damp weather.

Note: Cinnamon tends to encourage menstruation, so it should not be used excessively, or taken as a tea, during pregnancy.

Preparing and Using: Cinnamon can be bought whole in sticks or 'quills', or in powdered form. Both are useful; the quills have a better flavour and keep longer, but they are difficult to grind at home.

A little cinnamon stick can be added to an ordinary pot of weak tea for a delicious brew; or you could make the spiced tea described under ginger (page 60).

Cinnamon makes a delicious flavouring for both sweet and savoury dishes, and combines well with many fruits, vegetables and pulses. Add a piece of cinnamon stick to rice when you are cooking it; add a pinch or two of powdered cinnamon to fruit salads, or a piece of cinnamon stick to fresh or dried fruits, when you are stewing them. See the recipes for FIGS WITH PRUNES, PEARS AND APPLES (page 186) and COMPOTE OF QUINCES AND FIGS (page 200). Sprinkle powdered cinnamon over wholewheat toast, plain natural yogurt or fruit salad; add it to cakes and biscuits.

Essential oil of cinnamon is very hot, so it should be doubly diluted before use (see page 45).

CLOVES *Eugenia caryophillata*

Hot, tonic, antiseptic, raises the yang

The dried, unopened flower buds of a tropical tree, cloves have a pungent, sweet, astringent flavour and are digestive and aromatic.

Like mint, rosemary, fennel and ginger, cloves are helpful for those with cold constitutions and SLOW DIGESTIONS, cold abdomen, flatulence, hiccups and other evidence of putrefaction such as bloated stomach and heavy breath.

Other symptoms associated with coldness and low vitality respond well to cloves; they can strengthen a WEAK BACK and help mild impotence, or what the Chinese call WEAK YANG OF THE KIDNEYS. For this purpose cloves mix well with other warming spices such as ginger and cinnamon.

Cloves are a powerful antiseptic, capable of inhibiting viruses and fungi. This quality, combined with their warming, toning nature, makes them particularly useful for COLDS AND FLU. Used during the winter months, cloves can be a good preventative; they are helpful in the initial, 'shivery' stages of a cold or cough, good for clearing phlegm and blocked sinuses. Cloves are also an effective expectorant, helpful for BRONCHITIS and COUGHS, and for clearing mucus from the respiratory system.

Throughout the ages cloves have been known as a good remedy for gum and tooth infections where a powerful antiseptic action is required (see TEETH AND GUM PROBLEMS, page 217).

Preparing and Using: Cloves can be bought whole or ground; whole cloves have the best flavour, but are difficult to reduce to a powder.

For clove tea, infuse 2–3 cloves in a cup of freshly boiled water for 10 minutes. Just 2–3 cloves add flavour to a whole dish; try adding them to rice, before cooking, or to apples, quinces, pears and dried fruits when baking or poaching them. Cloves also go well with onions, beetroot, cabbage and carrots.

As the essential oil is quite strong, it needs to be well diluted: 3 drops is plenty in a bath; 2 drops in a saucer of oil, or make up a double-dilution massage oil.

CORIANDER *Coriandrum sativum*

Neutral to warming, digestive, tonic

Both the seeds and the leaves of coriander are useful. The leaves look and taste a little like flat-leaf parsley, which belongs to the same family, but coriander has a more citrus flavour. The seeds are rather like peppercorns – light brown, greenish or whitish in colour, with a mild, warm flavour, reminiscent of orange peel.

Coriander seeds act mainly on the digestive system where they assist the downward movement of energy, or digestive peristalsis. The seeds are strongly anti-spasmodic, so they ease abdominal cramps as well as allaying putrefaction in the stomach and intestines. This is an excellent remedy, therefore, for acute and chronic INDIGESTION when there is bloating, soreness, hiccups, belching, flatulence and cramps. As a secondary action, coriander seeds relieve HEADACHES due to digestive disturbances, and are reputed to increase vitality, especially when this is sapped through chronic indigestion.

The leaves of coriander have a similar, but weaker, action. They are more cooling and richer in vitamins and minerals. The essential oil of coriander seeds can be added to sunflower or almond oil and used to massage the abdomen, relieving pain due to indigestion.

Preparing and Using: Whole and ground coriander seeds are available; the whole seeds are easy to crush in a pestle and mortar or to powder in a coffee grinder. Fresh coriander is becoming more widely available; Middle Eastern shops are a good source. Both the seeds and the fresh leaves can be used to make tea in the usual way, and both are also useful in cooking.

Ground coriander, with its mild flavour, is a basic ingredient in many Middle Eastern dishes and in curries, where it is used generously to thicken as well as flavour. Coriander seeds and leaves are excellent with pulses and enhance many vegetables; they can be used together, the ground or crushed seeds being added at the beginning of cooking, the leaves snipped generously over the finished dish.

Coarsely crushed seeds can be stir-fried in olive oil with cabbage, carrots, mushrooms, aubergines, celery, fennel, courgettes or green beans and a little tomato purée and lemon juice to serve them *à la Grecque* (see the recipe for FENNEL À LA GRECQUE on page 112). Coriander seeds are also good cooked with apples.

FENNEL *Foeniculum vulgare*

Warm, dry, diuretic

Fennel is one of the most valuable plants in kitchen pharmacy, yielding a bulb which is delicious as a vegetable; feathery, fresh-tasting leaves; and seeds which are one of the oldest and most widely used spices, mentioned in ancient texts from Egypt, Greece, India and China. All parts of the plant have a warm, slightly sweet, liquorice flavour, and have a similar effect on the body; the seeds have the strongest action. Extensive research by nineteenth- and twentieth-century doctors, including Cadeac, Meunier, Cazin, Bodard, Bontemps, Coze and Valnet, has confirmed the therapeutic value of this plant.

Fennel moves the energy of the stomach and intestines, clears the lungs, eliminates water and tonifies the yang. The research of Cadeac and Meunier (1899) has shown that fennel seeds increase the general body tone and speed up the metabolic processes. Their main area of action is in the digestive tract, relieving symptoms of SLOW DIGESTION: abdominal swelling, hiccups, flatulence, heavy breath and CONSTIPATION. As Chinese laboratory tests have shown, they ease the functions of the gastro-intestinal tract, speeding digestion and encouraging the passing of wind. Fennel seeds have also been shown to relieve intestinal spasms, thus indicating their usefulness in complaints such as IRRITABLE BOWEL SYNDROME. In one recent study in China, 22 out of 26 patients with ulcerated hernias were helped by taking fennel seeds.

Another property of fennel seeds is that they help the digestive system to eliminate fats, thus inhibiting or preventing the production of mucus; and they also have an expectorant action, enabling the lungs to get rid of phlegm. In addition, fennel seeds have a marked diuretic quality, helping to eliminate OEDEMA (FLUID RETENTION). These qualities, the capacity to help the body get rid of fat and excess water, and also to ease constipation, make fennel seeds one of the most helpful aids to WEIGHT LOSS.

Throughout the ages fennel seeds have been considered valuable in increasing LACTATION. Fennel also has the reputation of improving the EYESIGHT, especially in people with poor digestion. In 1156 Hildegard of Bingen wrote about fennel seeds: 'Eaten daily on an empty stomach, they reduce mucus and all soreness, take away halitosis and clear the eyes.'

Note: Fennel seeds tend to encourage menstruation and therefore should not be taken frequently or in large doses during pregnancy. However, the bulb and leaves can still be eaten.

Preparing and Using: The seeds can be bought ground, but the whole ones are best and are soft enough to eat without grinding.

Fennel seeds can be taken as a tea, made in the usual way by infusing ½ teaspoon seeds in a cup of boiled water for 5–10 minutes. They can also be used as a tincture; the dosage is 15 drops in a little water 2–3 times a day.

Two or three drops of essential oil of fennel seeds can be mixed in a saucer of massage oil and some of this mixture can be regularly gently massaged over the abdomen. In the case of CONSTIPATION, the oil should be massaged along the large intestine, in a clockwise direction, for a few minutes.

Like aniseed, the liquorice flavour of fennel seeds complements many vegetables, including pulses. Cabbage, carrots, celery, courgettes, cucumber, leeks, spinach and onions are all enhanced by fennel seed, and a mixture of the bulb and seed is excellent (see the recipe on page 112).

Fennel seed can be used with some fruits. In Italy it is sometimes cooked with dried figs; and apples, pears, plums and quinces respond well to this flavouring, too. The bulb can be eaten raw, steamed, baked, sautéed or stir-fried (see the recipes on pages 110–13 fresh fennel fronds can be chopped into salads or sprinkled over cooked vegetables. In India roasted fennel seeds are eaten after a meal, as a digestive and breath-freshener.

GARLIC *Allium sativum*

Hot, antiseptic, expectorant

Garlic, a segmented bulb with a potent onion flavour, is renowned worldwide, both as a flavouring and as a medicine. Its use in ancient Egypt was documented 4500 years ago when a clove of garlic was given each day to the workers building the Pyramids to keep up their energy and ward off contagious diseases such as flu and colds. The famous Greek physician, Galen, called garlic 'the great panacea'.

The antiseptic action of garlic is effective against viruses, fungi and bacteria, and has been thoroughly researched and documented in both the West and East. This, combined with its power as an expectorant and its warming and strengthening action on the respiratory system, makes garlic extremely valuable in treating COLDS AND FLU when there is chilliness and shivering; it is also recommended for BRONCHITIS, COUGHS and ASTHMA with thick and persistent mucus.

In India and China, researchers have discovered the value of garlic in treating amoebic and similar types of DYSENTERY, killing the bacteria which cause these diseases. Garlic can be used in a similar way against many other organisms, including CANDIDA. For this action, the purple-skinned variety is recommended.

Garlic helps to eliminate harmful bacteria created by putrefaction of food in the gut due to a SLOW DIGESTION. It also has a vaso-dilatory action, increasing circulation, warming cold limbs, lowering HIGH BLOOD PRESSURE and helping to unclog blocked arteries in ATHEROSCLEROSIS and other conditions.

When using it for treatment, take 1 garlic clove twice a day with lunch and dinner for up to 3 weeks.

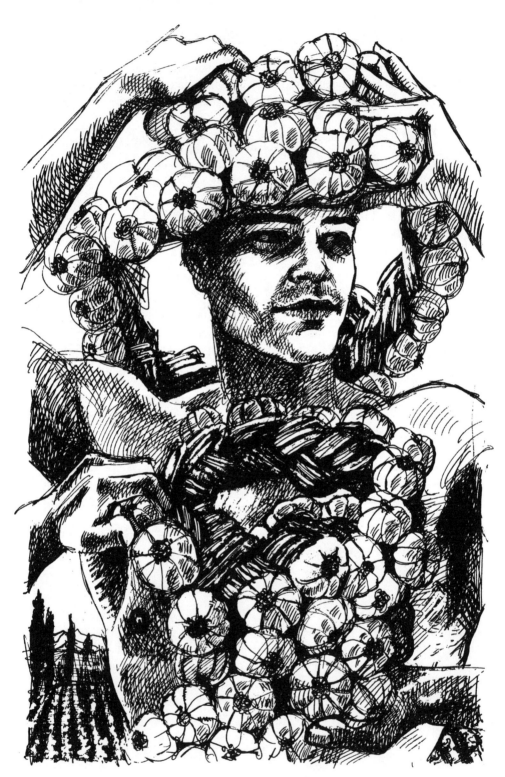

Crowns of braided garlic, Piedmonte

Note: Garlic should not be taken when there is an excess of heat or inflammation in the body, especially in the digestive system, as in GASTRITIS or ULCERS.

Preparing and Using: Powdered garlic and garlic salt are available but lack the flavour and qualities of fresh garlic. Garlic capsules are available from healthfood shops and chemists; the type made from freeze-dried garlic are best; hot-pressed oil of garlic is not as effective, as the garlic can lose some of its properties in the processing.

For an antibiotic action, eat 1 clove of garlic with your lunch and dinner for 2 weeks. Alternatively, you can take 2 freeze-dried capsules at each of these meals. For other purposes, the dosage is 1 clove of garlic a day. If you're worried about the effect of garlic on your breath, try chewing a little parsley or a cardamom pod and hope for the best!

The flavour of garlic enhances most savoury dishes. In fact, if you like garlic, it is easy for it to become a kitchen basic, used with almost as much regularity as salt and pepper. As a cure, garlic is more effective if taken raw; try chopping or crushing it and adding it to favourite salad vegetables or to vegetables which have already been cooked; rub a cut clove of garlic over hot toast, then dribble a little olive oil on top and serve with soups, salads and dips; add crushed garlic to cooked pasta or grains; or mash it with butter and serve with baked potatoes. Garlic also goes well with most pulses, especially chickpeas. See the recipes for EASY FELAFEL (page 140) and FAVOURITE HUMMUS (page 141).

GARLIC SOUP

This is a deliciously creamy soup. Although there is a lot of garlic in it, the flavour is quite mild, since the garlic is well cooked. This recipe can also be used to make an excellent non-dairy garlic sauce; the quantity given is enough for 4–6 people when made as a sauce. Serves 2.

> *225 g/8 oz potatoes, scrubbed and diced but not peeled*
> *2 garlic bulbs broken into cloves, but not peeled*
> *15 g/½ oz butter (optional)*
> *sea salt*

Put the potatoes in a pan with the garlic and 1.5 litres/2½ pints water. Cover and simmer for about 15 minutes, or until the potato is tender. Liquidise well, then pour through a sieve into a clean pan. Add a little more water if you want a thinner soup, then whisk in the butter, if using, and some salt to taste. Reheat gently before serving.

GERANIUM *Pelargonium odorantissimum*

Neutral to slightly cooling, yin tonic, astringent

Although the leaves of this fragrant plant can be used to perfume and flavour sweet dishes (see the recipe for PAWPAW WITH SCENTED GERANIUM LEAVES on page 194), the scented geranium is used mainly in the form of its essential oil which can help to calm NERVES, release TENSION and lift DEPRESSION. Whilst it is gently calming the nervous system, it is also strengthening the yin, so it is helpful when there are symptoms such as night sweats, tiredness and feverishness in the afternoon (see TOO LITTLE YIN, page 26).

Geranium has an anti-inflammatory and astringent quality, particularly when combined with essential oil of sandalwood. Diluted in a carrier oil such as sunflower or almond, and used to massage the lower abdomen gently in an anti-clockwise direction, these oils can help DIARRHOEA and GENITAL DISCHARGES. Geranium is also recommended for the hot flushes and night sweats of the MENOPAUSE; and it is considered to have a mildly tonic action on the pancreas, so it is useful for HYPO-GLYCAEMIA.

Preparing and Using: Geranium plants with edible, scented leaves can be grown in the garden and in window boxes. Their fragrance is delightful, and the leaves can be used to give a delicate, scented flavour to fruit salads and compotes, creams, fools, sorbets and ice-creams.

Essential oil of geranium can be put into a bath, or a few drops can be sprinkled on to a cotton handkerchief or on to your pillow. Added to a massage oil, either on its own or combined with another oil, such as lavender, it can be used to treat BURNS, ULCERS, INFLAMMATIONS and BITES. When used neat on a burner, or applied to the skin in a massage oil, geranium (like mint and lavender) is useful as an insect-repellent.

GINGER *Zingiber officinale*

Hot, dry

Ginger is a bulbous root with an aromatic, hot, slightly sweet flavour, and, when fresh, a definite citrus note which is lacking in the dried variety.

Along with other spices, such as fennel, mint and garlic, ginger has traditionally been used throughout the world as a culinary spice and therapeutic agent. Ginger is hot; it warms the stomach, raises the yang, moves the energy, improves the circulation of the blood, clears the lungs, and cures COLDS AND FLU.

Most plants act primarily on one area and have a secondary effect on others. Ginger, however, acts equally on many bodily functions to warm, tone and clear. It is extremely effective for colds and flu where there is shivering and a feeling of chilliness; it warms the body and promotes sweating.

Ginger is a powerful expectorant, useful when there is an accumulation of catarrh in the respiratory tract, as in colds or COUGHS with mucus and CONGESTED SINUSES, or BRONCHITIS and BRONCHIAL ASTHMA. As explained under MUCUS OR PHLEGM on page 29, whitish or transparent mucus denotes cold in the system (cold phlegm), and in this case the warming and expectorant qualities of ginger are strongly recommended. If the phlegm is deep yellow or green in colour, it means that there is heat in the system (hot phlegm), and in this case the heat of ginger needs to be regulated by cooling foods such as honey and lemon.

Ginger also has a very strong action on the digestive system. It is helpful for SLOW DIGESTION when the abdomen feels rather cold; for flatulence, belching and DIARRHOEA, especially if this follows the eating of very cold food. A recent report in the medical magazine *Anaesthetic* described the properties of ginger in reducing vomiting and nausea (quoting statistical evidence). This also confirms that ginger is one of the best remedies for TRAVEL SICKNESS.

As it increases the flow of blood to the extremities, ginger is very helpful for cold hands and feet, when taken internally, in food or as a tea. It can also be taken externally: 3–4 drops of essential oil of ginger are added to a saucer of oil and massaged into the legs and arms. Massaging this oil over the spine, and the adrenal and kidney area of the back, restores vitality when the yang energy is depleted, or there is a feeling of tiredness and cold.

Ginger is also very useful in cases of COLD RHEUMATISM, where there is a cold, cramping pain and swelling in the joints, aggravated by cold, damp weather. For this, ginger can be taken both externally and internally: a ginger bath is especially good.

Note: Laboratory research in China has shown that ginger can increase blood pressure, so it should not be used where there is HYPERTENSION or where there is excessive heat, inflammation and dryness of the system. Like aniseed, ginger should always be taken in moderation.

Preparing and Using: Fresh ginger is widely available and will keep for several weeks in the salad compartment of the fridge. Ground dried ginger which is even easier to obtain, is also worth keeping; and crystallised and preserved ginger are sometimes useful, although both contain white sugar.

For a ginger bath, add 15 g/½ oz of the crushed, fresh root, or 1 teaspoon ground dried ginger, to the running water. Don't add more than this, as higher quantities could cause burning and reddening of the skin.

To make ginger tea, boil a pinch of the powder or crushed root in a cupful of water for 5 minutes. This tea can be taken as it is, or used to brew tea leaves in the usual way. Other warming spices such as cinnamon and cloves can also be added, to make an aromatic, pleasant-tasting tea which will shorten the duration of a cold, or help to prevent one during the winter months. Alternatively, try taking ginger as a tincture: 5–10 drops of the tincture in a glass of water or fruit juice. It's best not to take this more than once or twice a day, and if you get a feeling of burning in your stomach, try reducing the dosage, or, if it persists, stop it altogether.

Fresh ginger can be added to many vegetables to bring the benefit of its warming therapeutic action as well as to add interest and flavour. Simply grate off as much ginger as you need from the root without peeling it, then keep the rest of the root in the fridge (rather like grating cheese). A teaspoonful will flavour a dish for 4 people delicately; a tablespoonful or more will give a stronger flavour and make the mixture hotter. Fresh ginger goes well with aubergine, pumpkin, potatoes, onions, leeks, cabbage, carrots, celery and courgettes. It can be added to soups, stir-fries, sautées and casseroles, as well as to rice and pulse dishes.

Ground ginger can be added to bread, biscuits, cakes and puddings; try some sprinkled over plain natural yogurt or stewed fruit, or add ginger to fruits before stewing, for a delicately spicy, warming dessert.

HONEY PARKIN

This sticky, wholesome cake – rich in iron and warmly flavoured with ginger – makes a nourishing treat for cold weather. Makes 12 pieces.

> *100 g/4 oz medium oatmeal*
> *100 g/4 oz plain wholewheat flour*
> *2–3 teaspoons ground ginger*

2 teaspoons baking powder
100 g/4 oz black treacle or molasses
100 g/4 oz clear honey
100 g/4 oz Barbados sugar
120 ml/4 fl oz very light olive oil or sunflower oil
120 ml/4 fl oz water or milk
50 g/2 oz flaked almonds

Set the oven to 180°C/350°F/Gas Mark 4. Line a 20 cm/8 in square tin with greaseproof paper. Put the oatmeal, flour, ground ginger and baking powder into a bowl. Gently warm the treacle or molasses, honey, sugar and oil until blended, then remove from the heat and add the water or milk. Add this mixture to the dry ingredients, mixing quickly and thoroughly. Pour the mixture into the prepared tin and sprinkle with the flaked almonds. Then bake for about 30 minutes, or until risen and lightly browned, when a skewer inserted into the centre comes out clean. Leave to cool in the tin and cut into pieces when cold.

HORSERADISH *Cochlearia armoracia*

Hot, stimulant, antiseptic

Horseradish is a long, thin root which tastes and, once cut, smells, like very hot watercress. The vapours can make your eyes water, as onions do. The properties of horseradish are similar to those described for other types of radish (see page 126). Horseradish is, however, hotter than the other radishes and, in herbal medicine, is mostly used as a stimulant for cold constitutions with poor circulation and weak energy. It is well-known for its effective action on COLDS when there is a feeling of chilliness and shivering. And it is a powerful expectorant, highly recommended for BRONCHITIS and blocked SINUSES. Horseradish is also helpful for COLD RHEUMATISM.

Note: Horseradish should not be taken when there is an excess of heat or inflammation in the body, especially in the digestive system, as in GASTRITIS or ULCERS.

Preparing and Using: Powdered, granulated and ready-grated forms of horseradish are available, although a whole horseradish root will keep for several weeks in the fridge and it is probably best to take it freshly grated. Simply trim and scrub or scrape the root, then grate it, avoiding the hard central core.

Try adding grated horseradish to yogurt or soured cream to make a sauce or dressing, or as a topping for jacket potatoes. Add a little to sandwiches; try cooked beetroot with an apple and horseradish sauce.

LAVENDER *Lavandula spica; Lavandula vera (officinalis)*

Neutral to slightly warming, analgesic, antiseptic, beneficial for the nerves

Lavender, with its familiar spiky green leaves and fragrant purple flowers, rates very highly amongst garden plants for its healing, calming and regenerating qualities. It is used mainly in the form of the essential oil, which, either on its own, or combined with other essential oils, has many uses.

Mixed with a carrier oil such as almond or sunflower and massaged over the joints, lavender can relieve the pain of ARTHRITIS; massaged twice a day over the bladder area, it can speed recovery from CYSTITIS and improve other genito-urinary infections such as NON-SPECIFIC URETHRITIS and THRUSH. On its own, or combined with essential oils of camomile and geranium, and massaged over the affected areas, lavender can ease pain from inflamed nerves, as in SCIATICA and TRIGEMINAL NEURALGIA (inflammation of the facial nerves). And, again, on its own, or with other essential oils, lavender can soothe TENSION, improve sleep and relieve HEADACHES when massaged over the shoulders, neck, forehead and temples.

For a strongly sedative and analgesic action, drink lavender tea.

Preparing and Using: A few lavender plants make an attractive addition to a garden and the flowers can be picked and dried; they can also be bought from herbalists.

To make lavender tea, add ¼ teaspoon dried lavender flowers to a cup of freshly boiled water, and infuse for 5 minutes. Drink this tea for no more than 10 days, then have a break of 10 days before continuing.

Add a few drops of essential oil of lavender to the bath, for relaxation and relief from pain.

Not only relaxing and analgesic in action, but also strongly antibacterial, antiseptic and healing, essential oil of lavender can be used in a much more concentrated form than usual for first aid purposes: a mixture of 20 drops essential oil to 2 teaspoons massage oil or ointment can be applied to BURNS, CUTS, BRUISES and BITES. In cases of emergency it can also be applied neat to such conditions.

Bunches of dried lavender in the home will discourage insects, as will burning the essential oil neat on a burner.

LEMON THYME *Thymus citriodorus*

Neutral, expectorant, antiseptic

A lemon-scented plant, with small green leaves, lemon thyme has the same properties as common thyme (see page 83) except that it is cooler. Lemon thyme is therefore useful for COLDS AND FLU where there is heat and feverishness; or for people who need the qualities of thyme but in a cooling form. The expectorant and mild anti-spasmodic properties of lemon thyme are helpful for clearing an accumulation of hot mucus (see page 220), in COUGHS, BRONCHITIS or ASTHMA.

Preparing and Using: Tea can be prepared in the usual way with ¼–½ teaspoon dried lemon thyme to a cupful of boiled water. The essential oil can be added to the bath (5–6 drops) or diluted in massage oil and rubbed gently over the throat, chest and back.

Like common thyme, lemon thyme is a useful herb in the kitchen, harmonising with, and enhancing, the flavour of most vegetables; it's also excellent with pulses and grains, and delicious in stuffings and casseroles.

LEMON VERBENA *Lippia citriodora*

Cooling, slightly drying, digestive, beneficial for the nerves

These long, slim, pointed leaves have a strong and pleasing lemon scent and flavour. Lemon verbena helps INDIGESTION and soothes the nervous system; it also calms STAGNANT ENERGY IN THE LIVER AND DIGESTION which creates a bitter taste in the mouth, digestive HEADACHES, bloating, belching, flatulence and ACIDITY. It has a mild action in helping the body to excrete phlegm from the digestive system – evidence of this can be a greasy tongue and mucus in the stools. For this purpose, lemon verbena combines very well with mint and fennel.

Lemon verbena, particularly if taken as a tea, which is probably the most usual and pleasant way of enjoying this herb, eases TENSION and INSOMNIA.

Note: Like all calming herbs, if taken in excess, lemon verbena can cause lethargy and debility.

Preparing and Using: It is easy to grow, though you can usually buy it in the form of tea bags.

To make your own lemon verbena tea, infuse ½ teaspoon dried leaves, or 2–3 torn fresh leaves, in a cup of freshly boiled water.

Just 1–2 leaves can also be added, whole, to a milk pudding before baking (unless of course you are taking lemon verbena for a condition which is aggravated by milk produce). You can sprinkle greased cake tins with chopped lemon verbena before putting in the cake mixture, for a delicately flavoured cake. The leaves also make a delightful addition to potpourri mixtures.

M A R I G O L D *Calendula officinalis*

Neutral to slightly warming, soothing, regulates the gynaecological system, works against tumours and growths

These beautiful orange flowers which grace our gardens and homes also have the power to strengthen and heal our bodies. Marigold has been used for many centuries to help LYMPHATIC SWELLINGS, CYSTS, WARTS and both malignant and non-malignant growths. It can be taken internally as a tincture or tea, or applied externally in the form of calendula ointment. The ointment is widely used by chiropodists for warts and VERRUCAE.

Marigold soothes STAGNANT ENERGY IN THE LIVER (see page 213); and it has a strong anti-inflammatory and healing action on the digestive system, so it is useful for conditions such as ULCERS, GASTRITIS, COLITIS, DIVERTICULITIS, DIARRHOEA, HAEMORRHOIDS (PILES) and IRRITABLE BOWEL SYNDROME.

A great friend of the female reproductive system, marigold is included in most herbal combinations for gynaecological problems. The ointment also has a wonderfully soothing and healing action on sore nipples which most mothers experience when they first start breast-feeding. Just apply the ointment after each feed.

For viral growths like warts, many herbalists are now prescribing neat application of the essential oil of another variety of marigold, the African marigold called Tagetes.

Preparing and Using: Marigolds are easy to grow in gardens, tubs and window boxes. The fresh flowers can be picked and dried, or dried flowers can be bought from herbalists.

Either fresh or dried petals can be used to make tea; a few can also be added to vegetable dishes or brown rice for a pretty colour and rather spicy flavour.

The ointment is available from most healthfood shops.

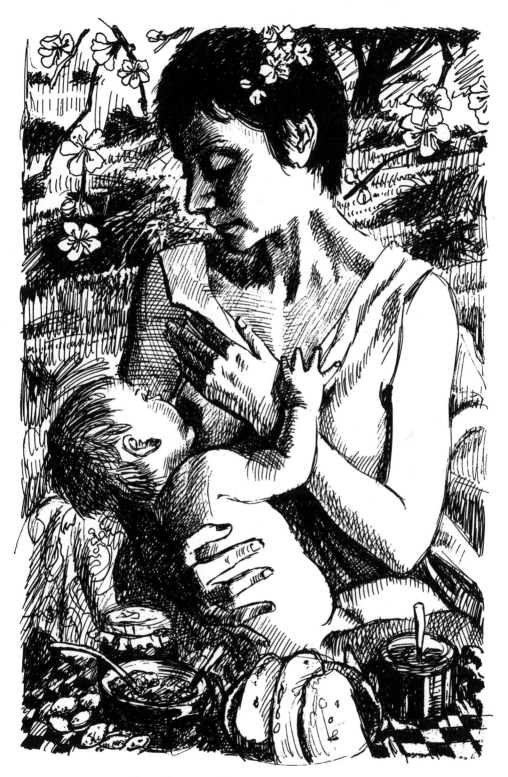

Almonds, oats and honey for the nursing mother

MARJORAM *Oreganum marjoram*

Neutral to warming, tonifying, relaxing, anti-spasmodic

Marjoram is a perennial plant with small, scented leaves. The flavour is sweet, warm and balmy.

There are many historical references to the beneficial uses of this herb: Dioscorides prescribed massages with an ointment of marjoram to warm and strengthen the nerves; Pliny used the herb for digestive cramps and belching; Mattioli, in the sixteenth century, for chest diseases with wheezing, oppression and mucus. In the Middle Ages, marjoram was frequently used as an ointment for rheumatic pains, paralysis with both flaccid and tense muscles, colds in the head and migraines.

Marjoram is both tonifying and relaxing, combining opposite qualities which work together to bring about balance and healing. Its primary action is on the nervous and respiratory systems, with a secondary action on the digestive system. The anti-spasmodic qualities of marjoram were demonstrated last century in the research of Cadeac and Meunier.

The toning/relaxing action of marjoram works on the nervous system to relieve TIREDNESS and TENSION in this way. Imagine a person who is over-active both physically and mentally. They drive themselves to the point of exhaustion, but cannot relax and rest because they are too tense, and the more tired they get, the more tense they become. If they take a tonic for the tiredness, the tension gets worse; yet if they try to calm the tension, they feel even more tired! This is where the dual action of marjoram is so helpful, for it both soothes and invigorates.

Marjoram has a similar effect on the lungs, soothing the distressing spasms of a COUGH or ASTHMA whilst at the same time helping to expel mucus and strengthening the respiratory system. In 1720, Dr Chomel, director of the medical department of the University of Paris, described marjoram as one of the best remedies for respiratory problems and COLDS with much sneezing. He also considered marjoram to be good for a tired, tense and forgetful brain (like rosemary and basil).

In the digestive system, marjoram eases spasms and COLITIS (like camomile). It also improves downward movement through the digestive system, eliminating putrefaction (like mint and fennel).

Marjoram is reputed to ease HEADACHES, especially when these are associated with nervous, respiratory or digestive problems, with symptoms of excessive or blocked energy, or lack of energy. According to folklore, marjoram can also calm excessive sexual ardour, especially if eaten with lettuce, either raw in a salad, or cooked, in a soup.

Preparing and Using: Marjoram tea is prepared in the usual way, using either fresh or dried herbs.

Fresh marjoram is good in salads; try it with tomatoes, instead of the more usual basil, or in a green salad. It's also good snipped over cooked vegetables, particularly carrots. Dried or fresh, marjoram makes a particularly pleasant addition to herb stuffings, along with thyme and parsley.

MINT *Mentha piperita*

Cooling, with warming potential, stimulant, anti-spasmodic, dry

Easily recognisable by its bright green colour and pungent aroma, mint has been used since ancient times in all major civilisations in both the East and the West. There are many types of mint growing throughout the world, but peppermint is the one which is best-known and most widely used medicinally. The easiest type of mint to use in the kitchen, however, is spearmint; the flavour of peppermint is rather strong for cooking, although excellent as a tea. These mints have very similar actions and either can be used.

According to Pliny, mint has a scent that awakens the spirit, and a flavour which stimulates the appetite. Laboratory tests in China have shown infusions of mint to be effective against echo viruses (which can cause respiratory and digestive problems) and salmonella typhi (which is the TYPHOID bacteria). In France studies by Sevelinges have shown it to be effective against STAPHYLOCOCCUS INFECTION, and studies by Courmont, Morel and Rochaix have revealed its efficacy against TUBERCULOSIS.

One of the most interesting properties of mint is that although it has a warming, pungent aroma and effect on the body at first, this later becomes refreshing and cooling.

COLDS AND FLU — both of the hot, feverish type and the cold, shivery kind — respond well to mint, and it eases stuffiness in the head and soreness in the eyes. Mint is helpful for SORE THROATS, too, perhaps combined with sage, as a tea; or in the form of the essential oil, mixed with massage oil and rubbed gently into the throat area. This oil also helps to draw out RASHES (such as MEASLES), in the early stages, thereby speeding recovery. The nervous system responds mildly to mint, which, rather like marjoram, induces relaxation but at the same time increases vitality.

Mint has a marked action on the liver and digestive system, and can be used to ease COLIC, flatulence, cramps, belching, hiccups, NAUSEA and digestive HEADACHES. For this, mint makes a pleasant after-dinner tea, and can be combined with other digestives such as fennel and aniseed.

Preparing and Using: Mint is easy to grow and several types of fresh mint can be bought during the summer. Dried mint is widely available and useful in winter, although, like basil, it loses much of its character in the drying process.

To make mint tea, use either ¼–½ teaspoon dried mint to a cup of freshly boiled water, or a good sprig of fresh mint, chopped or whole and lightly crushed. This tea is also good cold, or chilled, in hot weather.

The essential oil can be added to the bath. Or you could mix it with a base oil and massage it over the body: on the abdomen for INDIGESTION; on the chest and upper back for COLDS and respiratory problems; on the throat for SORE THROATS.

Mint can be used to flavour a whole range of dishes. It's good chopped fresh and sprinkled over many fruit salad mixtures; stirred, with honey, into natural yogurt; or added to home-made ice-cream. Mix it with sliced ripe Comice pear, as a first course or salad; snip it into salads, or over buttered new potatoes, carrots, cabbage or courgettes. Generous amounts of chopped mint, combined with parsley if you wish, can be forked into cooked rice; served cold, this mixture makes a refreshing salad. Perhaps one of the easiest and nicest ways of eating mint is in the form of MINT SAUCE (see below).

MINT SAUCE

This sauce goes as well with cooked beans and lentil burgers as it does with roast lamb. Serves 2–4.

> 8–10 *good sprigs of fresh mint*
> 2 *tablespoons apple juice concentrate*
> 1 *tablespoon wine vinegar or cider vinegar*

This is quickly made in a food processor: just remove any hard stems from the mint, then put everything into the processor with 2 tablespoons boiling water, and whizz until combined. Otherwise chop the mint, put into a small bowl, add the boiling water, then the apple juice concentrate and vinegar.

MUSTARD *Brassica alba; Brassica juncea; Brassica nigra*

Hot, expectorant, stimulant

These small, round seeds have a sharp, fiery flavour.

Being hot, mustard warms the stomach and abdomen, speeding a SLOW DIGESTION. It brings vitality as its heat surges through the body. Mustard is good for COLDS and COUGHS: its expectorant qualities help to clear mucus from the chest; and it is also good to take in the early stages of a cold when you feel chilly and under-par. In addition it increases circulation and warms COLD LIMBS.

Note: Mustard should not be taken when there is an excess of heat or inflammation in the body, especially in the digestive system, as in GASTRITIS or ULCERS.

Preparing and Using: Ground mustard is available as the familiar golden yellow powder. Or you can buy the whole seeds – black, white or brown. (Any colour can be used for most cooking purposes.) And there are also made-up mustards of various types.

Yellow powdered mustard can be added to a bath or foot-bath to increase the circulation and bring warmth. Use 2 teaspoons mustard powder to a foot-bath or 2–3 teaspoons to a normal bath.

A poultice of mustard powder can be applied to the chest to help clear congestion, mucus and coughs. Mix mustard powder to a thick paste with water; spread on a piece of gauze or cheesecloth and apply with the cloth next to the skin. Cover with another piece of fabric or an old towel.

Oil of mustard, which is a type of cooking oil, not an essential oil, can be bought from Indian, Bengali and Pakistani shops and massaged vigorously on the body and limbs. Indian wrestlers like to rub mustard over their bodies because it makes them feel warm and they believe it increases their strength and courage.

You can add whole mustard seeds to vegetable dishes (such as cabbage, carrot and cauliflower), giving them a hot, spicy flavour and pleasantly crunchy texture, and they are often used this way in Indian cookery. If you take the seeds as a tea, however, they can sometimes cause vomiting.

Try spreading a thin layer of made-up mustard on bread instead of butter when making sandwiches, or make a thick mustardy dressing for salad by whisking together 1 tablespoon made-up Dijon mustard, 1 tablespoon wine vinegar or lemon juice, 3 tablespoons light olive oil and salt and pepper to taste.

NUTMEG, MACE *Nux moscata, Myristica*

Warm, tonic

Nutmeg is the nut-like seed found in the fruit of a large tree; mace is the fleshy casing which surrounds it. Both nutmeg and mace have a warm, nutty, pleasantly bitter taste; medicinally, too, they have similar properties. They are general warming tonics, useful for people with a bloated, SLOW DIGESTION, low yang energy and a cold and lethargic constitution. They can also be of help when there is chronic DIARRHOEA due to a weak constitution. Both nutmeg and mace improve the circulation and bring warmth to COLD LIMBS.

Note: Nutmeg and mace can be toxic if taken in their more concentrated forms, so they should not be used as essential oils or in teas or tinctures. These spices tend to encourage menstruation so they should be avoided during pregnancy or if periods are heavy.

Preparing and Using: Both nutmeg and mace can be bought whole or ground. It's always worth buying whole nutmeg and grating it yourself. As mace is too hard to grind at home, the powder is more useful, although the whole pieces or 'blades' can be infused in liquid to draw out their flavour when this is appropriate in a recipe.

They are best used to flavour food, and are excellent grated or sprinkled over cooked cabbage, carrots, courgettes, pumpkin, mashed potatoes and spinach; or on top of creamy soups, such as potato, leek or onion. They're good in cakes and biscuits, too, or grated over milk puddings or custard, to make an aromatic topping.

OREGANO *Oreganum vulgare*

Warming, tonic, expectorant, digestive

The leaf of a sprawling perennial plant which grows wild in Mediterranean countries, oregano has a strong, warm, savoury flavour which survives drying unusually well.

Oregano has a powerful action on both the respiratory and digestive systems. Its natural antibiotic action, like that of thyme and cloves, can help clear RESPIRATORY INFECTIONS, especially if they produce a great deal of mucus and the patient feels chilly. Oregano eases COLDS AND FLU of the cold, shivery type rather than those with a fever. It also has a mild antispasmodic action which helps soothe COUGHS.

Like mint, rosemary and thyme, oregano facilitates the digestive process, removing putrefaction which can cause HALITOSIS (BAD BREATH), abdominal swelling, hiccups and belching.

Oregano is a good tonic, raising the yang energy in those who have cold constitutions with frequent respiratory infections, colds and weak digestion.

The essential oil is highly antiseptic. It can be used for genito-urinary problems such as CYSTITIS, THRUSH, GENITAL DISCHARGES and NON-SPECIFIC URETHRITIS, as well as for respiratory and digestive problems.

Preparing and Using: Essential oil of oregano is extremely hot, so it should be doubly diluted before use (see page 45).

For oregano tea, infuse ¼–½ teaspoon dried oregano, or a sprig of fresh oregano, in a cupful of freshly boiled water for 5 minutes.

Oregano is an easy herb to use in the kitchen, because its flavour enhances many savoury dishes. It is the usual herb with which to flavour pizza and gives a characteristically Italian flavour to any dish. Try it in tomato sauce, pasta dishes, beans and lentils, soups and casseroles.

PARSLEY *Petroselinum*

Neutral to cooling, stimulant, diuretic, nutritive

There are a number of varieties of this familiar bright green plant, all with mild, fresh-tasting leaves.

Parsley is a slight stimulant and tonic, partly because of its high vitamin and mineral content. It cleanses and enriches the blood which helps the skin, making this a useful herb for skin disorders such as ACNE and ECZEMA. It is also helpful for ANAEMIA.

The diuretic properties of parsley ease OEDEMA (FLUID RETENTION); while its high iron content, combined with oestrogen-like substances and its ability to increase menstrual flow, make this an especially helpful herb for weak anaemic women with scanty periods. The cleansing, diuretic qualities of parsley are also valuable for RHEUMATISM; and it can help digestion and increase the flow of bile.

Note: Because it increases the menstrual flow, parsley should not be taken in the form of tea during pregnancy or by women with heavy periods, although it can still be used as a flavouring in foods.

Preparing and Using: Parsley loses much of its flavour during the drying process; fresh parsley is undoubtedly best for cooking, although dried parsley can be used for making tea: ¼–½ teaspoon to a cupful of freshly boiled water, infused for 5 minutes.

There are numerous ways in which parsley can be used in cooking; this versatile herb combines with practically all vegetables and is particularly good chopped and added, in generous amounts, with butter, after cooking. It's also refreshing in salads; try it in TABBOULEH (see below).

For a parsley soup, follow the recipe for WATERCRESS SOUP (page 136) but instead of watercress, use a large bunch of fresh parsley; you could also try adding plenty of parsley to POLENTA (page 156). Old-fashioned parsley sauce is another good way of using this herb; make a béchamel or white sauce, then add chopped parsley until the mixture looks really green and tastes fresh.

TABBOULEH

The basis of this salad, bulgur wheat, sometimes called burghul, or pourgouri in Middle Eastern shops, is wheat which has been cracked and pre-cooked. The salad is refreshing yet substantial to eat; it's extra good when made several hours in advance so that the flavours have time to blend. Serves 2–3.

> 100 g/4 oz bulgur wheat
> salt
> 2 tablespoons olive oil
> 2 tablespoons fresh lemon juice
> 1 garlic clove, peeled and crushed
> 1–2 tablespoons finely chopped fresh mint
> 3 tablespoons finely chopped parsley
> 4 tomatoes, chopped
> 5 cm/2 in cucumber, diced
> ½ avocado, peeled and diced (optional)
> cos or other lettuce leaves, to serve

Put the bulgur wheat in a bowl with a good pinch of salt and cover with 150 ml/5 fl oz boiling water. Leave for 15 minutes, to allow the wheat to absorb the water. Then add the oil, lemon juice, garlic, mint and parsley. At this point the salad can be left in a cool place for up to 24 hours. Stir in the tomato and cucumber, and avocado if using, just before serving the salad. Serve on a base of lettuce leaves; these make good scoops for eating the salad.

PEPPER *Piper nigrum*

Hot, stimulant, circulatory, expectorant

Peppercorns are the fruit of a tropical plant; they may be green, white or black, depending on the stage at which they were picked. Black and green peppercorns are both the immature fruits; white peppercorns are the almost ripe fruits with their outer dark skins removed. The flavour is hot and pungent, black peppercorns being the most fiery, the others less so. Pink peppercorns come from another plant and are not related to the others.

Pepper is of course one of the most useful seasonings in the kitchen and so widely used as to be almost taken for granted. It does, however, have medicinal properties similar to those described for chillies (see page 51).

Note: Pepper should be used sparingly when a cooling diet is required, and people with LIVER PROBLEMS should eat pepper only occasionally.

Preparing and Using: Both black and white pepper are best when freshly ground, through a pepper mill, or, for a coarser texture, with a pestle and mortar. Both types of pepper are useful in the kitchen, white peppercorns being better in dishes in which a delicate, slightly sweet pepper flavouring is required.

A delicious mixture of the two types of pepper, coarsely ground, and called mignonette, is widely used in French cookery. Equal parts of black and white peppercorns and coriander seeds, ground together through a peppermill, also makes an excellent flavouring for almost any savoury dish.

Green peppercorns can be bought pickled in brine or vinegar; dried, or freeze-dried. The pickled ones should be rinsed well before adding to recipes; the dried ones can be ground like other peppercorns, or used whole after being soaked in water for a few minutes.

ROSE *Rosa damascena; Rosa gallica*

Cool, moist, yin tonic, regenerative, anti-inflammatory

Favourite flower of many, the rose has also always been a favourite natural remedy in countries as far apart as Egypt and India. It is most frequently used as a tea; as rosewater, a liquid made by steeping rose petals in water; as an essential oil, which is expensive but wonderful; and as a jam, which you can make from the dried or fresh petals (see recipe below).

Like geranium, rose can soothe and calm a hyperactive personality but at the same time strengthen and nourish the yin, relieving heat and inflammation while tonifying weak constitutions. (For the symptoms of TOO LITTLE YIN, see page 26.) Rose calms an OVERHEATED LIVER and cools the blood. It also cools the digestive system, helping both hot CONSTIPATION or DIARRHOEA and other diseases due to heat in the digestive tract. Again, both the tea, and the essential oil, massaged over the abdomen, are helpful for this, as they are for PREMENSTRUAL TENSION, DYSMENORRHOEA (PAINFUL PERIODS) and MENORRHAGIA (HEAVY MENSTRUAL BLEEDING). Both the essential oil, diluted in almond oil and applied externally, and the tea, taken internally, can regenerate and rejuvenate the skin.

Rose is believed to help WEAK YIN OF THE HEART (see page 246); it also soothes emotions which have been hurt through painful relationships, sorrow and guilt; the scent of roses comforts and cherishes the heart. Rose is reputed to increase fertility, affection and sexual desire in both men and women.

Preparing and Using: If you can grow or obtain petals from *Rosa gallica* or *Rosa damascena*, these are ideal, and can be used fresh or dry. The petals from some types of heavily scented red roses can be used; try them, and see what they are like. Many do not cook to a soft enough consistency for making rose petal jam. Cut off the white part at the base of the petals before using them. Dried rose petals can be obtained from herbalists, and ready-made rose petal jam from Indian shops.

To make rose petal tea, just put a few fresh or dried petals into a cup and add freshly boiled water.

The fresh petals can be added to fruit and vegetable salads, creams and ice-creams.

ROSE JAM

This jam not only tastes delicious, but also has valuable therapeutic qualities, helping to heal BRONCHIAL AND RESPIRATORY CONDITIONS. It can be eaten from the spoon or spread on bread, and makes a delicious topping for thick yogurt or vanilla ice-cream. This recipe has no added sugar and makes a small amount of jam; the quantities can be increased. You can use either dried fragrant rose petals from a herbalist, or fresh petals from scented red roses. Whether dried or fresh, the rose petals should become tender. Buy the spread from health shops, and use a triple-distilled rosewater from Middle Eastern shops. Makes 450 g/1 lb.

> *25—40 g/1—1½ oz dried rose petals,*
> *or 50—75 g/ 2—3 oz fresh ones*
> *450 g/1 lb pear and apple pure fruit spread*
> *1 tablespoon rosewater*

Put the dried rose petals in a saucepan, cover with water and leave to soak for about 1 hour. If you are using fresh petals, wash them and cut out the white part at the base of each one. Simmer either dried or fresh petals in water to cover for up to 1 hour, or until the petals are tender and little or no water is left. (Keep an eye on the water level and top up if necessary during the cooking time.) Strain the rose petals, pressing them against the sieve to make them as dry as possible. Put them back in the saucepan and, over a low heat, stir in the pear and apple pure fruit spread. When thoroughly mixed, remove from the heat and add the rosewater. Bottle and store in the fridge.

ROSEHIPS AND HIBISCUS *Rosa canina; Hibiscus spp*

Cooling, tonic

Hibiscus and rosehips have a similar action. They are both generally taken in the form of tea, often together, a beautiful red liquid with a powerful healing action on the body. They have a high vitamin C content, helping COLDS AND FLU and strengthening the body's immune system and resistance to disease. They are a safe and effective diuretic, easing OEDEMA (FLUID RETENTION), and also cleansing the genito-urinary tract, useful in conditions such as CYSTITIS. They cool an OVERHEATED LIVER and an OVERHEATED STOMACH, and they soothe an IRRITATED COLON which gives rise to DIARRHOEA. They are also recommended for pain and SWELLINGS IN THE SPLEEN.

Both hibiscus and rosehips have a beneficial effect on CIRCULATORY PROBLEMS. In particular, they strengthen the walls of the capillaries and increase the elasticity of the arteries.

In areas of the Sudan where people drink a great deal of hibiscus tea, the incidence of CANCER is much lower than average. Research is being conducted to discover whether these two factors are linked.

Preparing and Using: Hibiscus and rosehips are best taken in the form of tea. You can buy them separately or mixed, in the form of teabags from healthfood shops, or as loose tea from herbalists. In Italy you can buy dried whole hibiscus flowers and you simply add 2–3 to a cupful of boiled water.

These teas are good chilled in the summer. Try making a pot of tea, then adding sliced fruit, such as strawberries, raspberries or peaches; leave to cool, then chill. Fragrant herbs and spices, such as mint leaves, cloves or cinnamon stick, can also be added, to vary the flavour and therapeutic properties of the brew.

R O S E M A R Y *Rosmarinus officinalis*

Warm to hot, tonic, moves the energy and circulation, raises the yang

These short spiky leaves of an aromatic Mediterranean shrub (now grown in many parts of the world) have a warm, aromatic flavour, redolent of pine, which survives the drying process well.

Celebrated in the poetry of Orazius (60 BC), and praised for its medicinal uses by early physicians such as Theophrastus, Dioscorides and Galen, rosemary was considered a sacred plant in ancient Greece and Rome. The dried leaves and essential oil of rosemary were also found in early Egyptian tombs.

Rosemary has a warming, moving and tonifying action. It has been used for thousands of years to warm, cleanse and move the energy of the liver. This remedy is recommended for people with a sluggish, COLD LIVER AND GALL BLADDER, symptoms of which are a pale, yellowish complexion, SLOW DIGESTION, bitter taste in the mouth and lack of vitality. To increase your vitality, massage essential oil of rosemary down your spine and over the kidney and adrenal areas. Because of its stimulating effect on the circulation, rosemary increases the flow of blood to the genital area and is therefore also considered to be an aphrodisiac.

Whether taken internally or externally, rosemary increases the circulation of the blood, warming COLD LIMBS, especially during the winter; it's particularly good for COLD RHEUMATISM.

Rosemary is said to sharpen the memory, probably by increasing the blood supply to the brain, and is a useful herb to take when preparing for examinations. NERVOUS WEAKNESS and DEPRESSION are also helped by rosemary, especially if caused by overwork and concentration.

In the Middle Ages sprigs of rosemary added to the bath water were considered rejuvenating, as was massaging the face with an infusion of the herb. To discourage wrinkles, add 2–3 drops essential oil of rosemary to 1 litre/1¾ pints warm water and use as a face wash first thing in the morning; then massage your face with a mixture of 10 drops essential oil of rosemary to 100 ml/3½ fl oz almond oil. This treatment is not suitable for red or inflamed skin. An infusion of rosemary, or the essential oil diluted in a massage oil, applied to the scalp, slows HAIR LOSS and adds lustre.

Note: Rosemary should not be used if you have HYPERTENSION (HIGH BLOOD PRESSURE), 'BURSTING' HEADACHES of a hot type, or any hot disease. Because it tends to encourage menstruation, rosemary should not be taken during pregnancy or if periods are heavy; and avoid taking it at night if you want to sleep.

Preparing and Using: Rosemary can be bought fresh or dried all year round. To make rosemary tea, add a small sprig of the fresh herb or a pinch of dried to a cupful of water just off the boil; infuse for 5 minutes.

For a rosemary bath, add 5–6 drops essential oil to a bath, or 4–5 drops to a foot-bath to help the circulation and ease rheumatic pain.

Rosemary massage oil is made by adding 4–5 drops essential oil to a saucer of almond or sunflower oil.

In cooking, the strong flavour of rosemary goes well with pulse dishes, and blends best with fairly bland vegetables such as cabbage, courgettes, pumpkin, carrots and potato, as well as aubergine. Try snipping tender fresh shoots of rosemary over freshly cooked, buttered vegetables, or into a bowl of mixed salad. Rosemary also harmonises with meats; it's traditionally used to flavour lamb, often with garlic.

Sprinkle dried rosemary over bread or savoury biscuits before baking; or add it to butter, spread it on slices of granary stick, put them back in the shape of a loaf, wrap in tin foil, and bake for 10–15 minutes until the butter has melted and the bread is crisp. Rosemary is also good added to cooked brown rice. This mixture can then be used as a stuffing for peppers, large tomatoes or aubergines. Or you could flavour a fruit salad by burying 1–2 sprigs of rosemary in a bowl of mixed sliced fresh and cooked fruits and honey.

SAGE *Salvia officinalis*

Neutral to slightly warm, tonifies both yin and yang

Sage is the long, pointed, green leaf of a shrubby plant, with an aromatic, rather resinous flavour, widely available in its dried form, and, increasingly, fresh. It is one of the most important remedies of Western kitchen pharmacy. It was used and valued in ancient Egypt, Greece and Rome, through the Middle Ages, to the present time. In the medieval Salernitan School (based in Salerno, Italy), it was said of sage: 'Cur moriatur homo, cui salvia crescit in horto?' – 'Why does the man in whose garden sage grows die?'

Sage strengthens the lungs; it is therefore useful for those who often feel weak and are prone to COUGHS, COLDS AND FLU, particularly if their symptoms include a SORE THROAT. In fact, sage is one of the best remedies for throat infections, used as a gargle or tea, or, in the form of the essential oil, massaged over the throat.

In the last century sage was used to help sufferers from TUBERCULOSIS, especially if their symptoms included night sweats, emaciation and swollen lymph glands. The fact that sage was helpful for these conditions suggests that it may strengthen the immune system. Today, sage is recommended for excessive sweating, particularly if this happens during the night, a sign of severe weakness. Sage speeds recovery in any debilitating disease and helps convalescence. It is one of the best remedies for NEURASTHENIA or NEUROSIS, weakness with POOR CONCENTRATION and DEPRESSION.

Sage helps the digestion, especially when the patient is weak and debilitated; being a tissue tonic, it has astringent qualities which can be helpful when there is chronic DIARRHOEA. Sage stimulates the adrenal glands if taken as a tea (see below) or, in the form of the essential oil, added to massage oil and rubbed over the lower back. This is also helpful for strengthening weak or flaccid limbs.

The presence of oestrogen-like substances means that sage has a beneficial effect on the female reproductive system, increasing fertility, easing AMENORRHOEA (OR LACK OF PERIODS), and sweating or hot flushes during the MENOPAUSE.

An infusion of sage, or the massage oil, perhaps with some rosemary and nettle, can be rubbed into the scalp to help counteract HAIR LOSS.

Note: Because it tends to encourage menstruation, sage should not be taken as a tea or used in the form of the essential oil during pregnancy or if periods are heavy, although it can be used as a flavouring in food. During lactation, sage can discourage the flow of milk.

Preparing and Using: To make sage tea, infuse a pinch of dried sage or 1–2 leaves of fresh sage, torn and bruised, in a cupful of just-boiled water. Flavour with a little lemon and honey if you like.

The strong flavour of sage means that it needs to be used sparingly in the kitchen. Sage complements onions particularly well, and also apples when used in savoury dishes.

For a satisfying vegetarian dish, try packing SAGE AND ONION STUFFING (see below) into a marrow; wrap in buttered paper, bake at 200°C/400°F/Gas Mark 6 for about 1 hour until tender, and serve with apple sauce. For another version of the sage–onion–apple theme, try cooking a chopped onion in oil, then adding a large chopped cooking apple, 225–350 g/8–12 oz cooked haricot beans and 1 teaspoon sage, and cooking with a lid on the pan until the apple has formed a purée.

Sage also goes well with cheese, as it does with any fatty food, since it cuts the richness.

SAGE AND ONION STUFFING

This makes a delicious filling for vegetables such as marrow, large open mushrooms, pumpkin and courgettes. Adjust the quantities as necessary.

> 1 *tablespoon chopped onion*
> 100 *g/4 oz soft wholewheat breadcrumbs*
> 1 *teaspoon sage*
> 1 *teaspoon thyme*
> 1 *teaspoon marjoram*
> 25 *g/1 oz butter*
> *sea salt and freshly ground black pepper*

Mix all the ingredients together, moisten with water if needed, season to taste with salt and pepper, and use to stuff the vegetable of your choice. This stuffing also goes well with goose, duck and pork.

SAVORY *Satureja spp*

Hot, tonic, aphrodisiac, digestive, expectorant, antiseptic

There are two main types of this perennial herb, summer savory and winter savory. Both have a hot, rather peppery flavour and a toning, stimulating action which is also highly antiseptic. Savory increases and warms the yang energy, and − like rosemary, sage and thyme − strengthens the adrenals and activates the brain.

Savory warms and speeds the digestion, relieving bloating, belching and flatulence due to SLOW DIGESTION and putrefaction in the digestive canal. Its warming qualities also make this herb helpful for COLDS when there is shivering and copious white mucus, and for BRONCHITIS of the cold type. Savory might be used for these conditions in conjunction with thyme, ginger and chillies. RESPIRATORY, DIGESTIVE and URINARY INFECTIONS all respond well to the warming, antiseptic properties of savory.

Essential oil of savory is extremely hot and therefore needs to be doubly diluted (see page 45). Rub the massage oil over the chest and corresponding areas of the back to ease chest conditions; over the abdomen, to help digestion; up the spine for vitality; on the lower back as an aphrodisiac; into the feet and hands to warm them and increase the circulation.

The aphrodisiac properties of savory have been renowned since ancient Greece. During the festival of Bacchus in Greece, the sacred sticks of the priests were decorated with savory to symbolise joy and pleasure.

Preparing and Using: Savory tea is made by infusing ½ teaspoon dried savory in hot water; it is best to take this not more than once a day; you certainly should not have more than 2 cups a day.

The peppery flavour of savory harmonises with many dishes. It is particularly good with beans and pulses and is known in Germany as 'the bean herb'.

TARRAGON *Artemisia dracunculus*

Neutral, digestive, anti-spasmodic

Tarragon is a bright green perennial herb with long, slim, pointed leaves and a markedly aniseed flavour. It is available both dried and fresh and acts mainly on the stomach and digestive system, speeding a SLOW DIGESTION, easing swelling and flatulence, soothing spasms and COLIC.

Like mint and basil, tarragon mildly stimulates but at the same time calms the nervous system, so it is particularly helpful for digestive upsets caused by STRESS and NERVOUS TENSION.

Note: As it tends to encourage menstruation, tarragon should not be used during pregnancy or when periods are heavy.

Preparing and Using: Add the essential oil of tarragon to the bath, or make it up into a massage oil and rub it on to the abdomen to soothe digestive upsets.

For tarragon tea, infuse ½ teaspoon dried tarragon or a good sprig of fresh, in a cupful of boiled water for 5–10 minutes.

Fresh tarragon is particularly good snipped into salads or over delicately flavoured cooked vegetables such as marrow, courgettes, cabbage, carrots or potatoes, or over creamy soups, such as potato soup; in omelettes; with fish or chicken. It also goes well with ripe Comice pears, to make a refreshing first course. Or you could try it in a salad made entirely of herbs. Mix fresh tarragon with several of the following: parsley, mint, chives, fennel, sorrel, chervil and marjoram, including a few of the flower heads if available. Dress with balsamic vinegar, or wine vinegar with a dash of honey.

THYME *Thymus vulgaris*

Hot, dry, tonic, antiseptic

There are many varieties of this aromatic, warming plant with its pungent flavour. It was widely used, both as a flavouring and as a medicine, by the ancient Egyptians, Greeks and Romans, who set great store by its healing properties. Modern studies by Campden, Cadeac and Meunier have demonstrated the effect of essence of thyme on the nervous system, whilst many researchers have found that essential oil of thyme is much more powerful than most antiseptics. In 1887 Chamberland found essential oil of thyme effective against ANTHRAX; in 1889 Cadeac and Meunier against TYPHOID; in 1922 Morel and Rochaix against, among other things, MENINGITIS and DIPHTHERIA; and recent research by Professor Novi in Italy has shown that thyme can activate and strengthen the immune system.

Thyme amplifies the heartbeat, increases the metabolic rate, cheers the heart and lifts the spirit. Like rosemary, thyme warms and tonifies; like cloves it is a powerful antiseptic and expectorant. This combination

83

of qualities means that thyme is excellent for COLDS of the shivery type, and for chronic and acute BRONCHITIS, helping the body to get rid of bacteria, strengthening and warming the lungs, expelling phlegm and clearing blocked sinuses. In fact thyme is useful for removing mucus from anywhere in the body.

With its ability to warm and tone, thyme is beneficial for anyone with low vitality, coldness, frequent infections and COLD LIMBS. Its powerful antiseptic action, capable of inhibiting many viruses and fungi, makes thyme valuable in treating genito-urinary complaints including CYSTITIS, THRUSH and GENITAL DISCHARGES.

Like rosemary, marjoram and oregano, thyme eliminates putrefaction in the abdomen and helps SLOW DIGESTION, especially in a cold, slow constitution. It is also reputed to improve the memory and brighten the hair, qualities which it shares with marjoram, rosemary, basil, mint and orange flowers.

Preparing and Using: Thyme is a herb which survives the drying process well, its flavour remaining much the same dried as fresh.

It makes a good tea, but it is strong; ¼–½ teaspoon dried thyme infused in a cup of freshly boiled water for 5 minutes is enough.

Essential oil of thyme is very hot and needs to be doubly diluted before use (see page 45). It can then be rubbed over the chest and lungs for RESPIRATORY AILMENTS; on the limbs for COLD EXTREMITIES and CHILBLAINS, and on the back for vitality.

Although pungent, thyme is quite a versatile herb, harmonising with most vegetables. It makes an excellent flavouring for pulse and grain dishes; for vegetable soups, stuffings and casseroles.

Vegetables

Like the grains, as well as being good to eat and having their own positive effect on the body, vegetables make a useful base for herbs and spices with their more concentrated flavours and intense action. They are of course packed with vitamins and fibre, and recent scientific research has shown that some vegetables can help protect us against certain forms of cancer. The target suggested by the World Health Organisation, as mentioned elsewhere in this book, is to eat at least 450 g/about 1 lb of fresh vegetables and fruit each day.

BUYING, STORING AND USING

Choose organically grown vegetables whenever possible; look for bright, fresh ones without signs of limpness. Store in a cool place; all vegetables except potatoes will keep well for several days in the fridge. Potatoes should be stored in a cool, dark place.

Trim the vegetables, cutting off any tough stems or inedible parts before using. It is not always necessary to peel root vegetables, especially if they have been organically grown. Just give them a good scrub; this conserves both the flavour and the nutrients. Leaf vegetables, especially spinach, need thorough washing in plenty of cold water; and all vegetables should be washed before use to remove any traces of pollutants.

Many vegetables are both delicious and nutritious eaten raw and you'll find recipe suggestions for salads throughout this section. According to Chinese medicine, salads are cooling, and therefore particularly useful during warm weather or when there are hot, inflammatory conditions in the body (see page 38 for details of the ANTI-INFLAMMATION DIET).

When cooking, most vegetables need only a few minutes until they are just tender. A steamer set over a saucepan of water is ideal; it also means that you can cook two vegetables at once, one in the steamer, and another – perhaps a leafy green vegetable – added later to the water below. When cooked, the vegetables can be tossed in butter, vegetable margarine or olive oil and flavoured with chopped herbs, spices, seasonings, and other ingredients, such as a squeeze of fresh lemon juice.

If your particular diet allows the use of some fat, other good ways of cooking vegetables are stir-frying and braising. For stir-frying you need a large saucepan or, preferably, a wok. Heat 1–2 tablespoons oil and put in the vegetables, which should be cut up into fairly small pieces. If you are stir-frying several vegetables, start with the vegetables which take the longest time to cook – onions and carrots, for instance – and add the others after a few minutes, stirring the mixture often. You can cover the pan and leave it over a low heat for a little while to help the harder vegetables to soften. Some flavourings, such as crushed garlic or grated fresh ginger, can be put in at the beginning of cooking; others, like fresh herbs, lemon juice, grated orange or lemon peel, and shoyu or tamari soy sauce are best added at the end.

Braising vegetables is similar to stir-frying in that you start by stirring them briefly in heated oil or melted butter; then they are cooked gently in a covered pan, with or without a little additional liquid, which is mainly absorbed during the cooking, resulting in tender vegetables in a natural sauce.

Simple vegetable soups are frequently used in kitchen pharmacy; they are easy to eat when you are feeling unwell and you will find a number of recipes for them in this section, including the CLEAR VEGETABLE BROTH below.

CLEAR VEGETABLE BROTH

You can vary this basic broth according to your whim and the ingredients available. It's nice with some whole garlic cloves added or a piece of leek or a few green beans; and other herbs, such as thyme or bay, either fresh or dried. Some grated fresh ginger is good, too. A dash of tamari, shoyu or miso can be added at the end, in which case you probably won't need salt. Serves 4.

> 4–5 *outer sticks of celery*
> 4 *carrots*
> *a few leaves of spinach*
> *a small bunch of parsley*
> *sea salt*

Chop all the ingredients finely and put them into a large saucepan with 1.2 litres/2 pints water. Bring to the boil, then cover and leave to simmer gently over a low heat for 20 minutes. Remove from the heat and leave until cool, then strain. Unless you want a really clear broth, you can press the vegetables against the sieve to extract as much goodness and flavour as possible; this will make the mixture a bit cloudy but more nutritious. Reheat, season to taste with salt, and serve.

ARTICHOKE, GLOBE *Cynara scolymus*

Cool, moist, nourishes the yin and the blood

This vegetable, widely used in Mediterranean countries but less so in Great Britain, not only tastes delicious but has many valuable properties.

Artichokes act mainly on the liver, gall bladder, kidneys and blood. They detoxify a congested OVERHEATED LIVER, the symptoms of which are hot flushes, red face, tension, irritability, bitter taste in the mouth, acidity, INDIGESTION and soreness in the sides. Artichokes also clean and cool OVERHEATED KIDNEYS, easing symptoms such as backache, dark urine and a burning sensation when urinating.

The moist quality of artichokes helps to increase the yin energy, the need for which is shown by slight feverishness in the afternoon, hot feet and soles, and night sweats. Their high mineral content makes them useful in ANAEMIA (or what the Chinese call EMPTY OR WEAK BLOOD) with a feeling of tiredness, and brittle nails and split hair.

Artichokes are a very effective laxative, encouraging intestinal peristalsis and moistening the intestines, thus helping the evacuation of dry stools, and improving chronic CONSTIPATION. The diuretic action of artichokes makes them valuable for WEIGHT LOSS, along with fennel and celery.

HOT RHEUMATISM – when there is heat and dryness in the joints – responds well to artichokes. Artichokes purify the blood, the need for which is shown by a hot, red and inflamed skin.

Eaten as part of a purifying diet, artichokes help to lower cholesterol levels in the blood, so they can be helpful for ATHEROSCLEROSIS and HYPERTENSION (HIGH BLOOD PRESSURE). They can be a minor help in cases of DIABETES and other imbalances of sugar metabolism such as HYPO- and HYPERGLYCAEMIA.

Note: Over-consumption of artichokes can reduce lactation in nursing mothers.

Preparing and Using: Cut the stalks and inedible leaves off the artichokes so that only the tender leaf-bases remain. Cut away the inner transparent leaves and carefully scrape out the hairy choke, being careful not to damage the heart. Sprinkle the cut surfaces with lemon juice to preserve the colour. Large artichokes need cooking for about 40 minutes, on top of the stove in enough water to cover them. Or you could put them in the oven at 200°C/400°F/Gas Mark 6 in a roasting tin with enough water to come halfway up the artichokes and a piece of foil to cover them. They are done when a leaf will pull off easily.

If you can get the delicious baby artichokes, you only need to discard the outer tough leaves, then halve or quarter them as necessary. These baby artichokes can be stewed in olive oil, with a lid on the pan, until they are tender. Drain well and serve with a little olive oil or melted butter and a tiny bit of salt. Add some crushed garlic to the butter or olive oil for a remedy which is still cleansing but less cooling. Cooked artichokes are also delicious served cold, with some vinaigrette dressing or fresh lemon juice and olive oil.

87

ARTICHOKE BROTH

The cooking water from artichokes can be used to make a broth which is helpful for WEIGHT LOSS. Make sure you cook the artichokes in a stainless steel or enamel saucepan – not aluminium, as this reacts with the artichokes. Serves 2–3.

> 2–3 *outside sticks of celery, chopped*
> 1 *small fennel, chopped*
> 1 *teaspoon fennel seeds*
> 1–2 *potatoes, scrubbed and roughly sliced (optional)*
> 2–3 *carrots, scraped and roughly chopped (optional)*
> 3–4 *whole garlic cloves, unpeeled (optional)*
> *sea salt (optional)*
> *chopped celery leaves or fennel leaves (optional)*

Save 1 litre/1¾ pints cooking water from the artichokes (make up the quantity with water if necessary). Put this in a saucepan with the celery, fennel and fennel seeds. Bring to the boil, cover and simmer for 20–25 minutes until the celery is very tender. For a slightly thicker soup, you can add the potatoes, carrots and garlic cloves, and simmer until all the vegetables are tender. Purée, then strain, and season with a little salt if your diet allows it. Fresh chopped celery leaves or fennel leaves can be added before serving for extra flavour and interest.

ARTICHOKE RICE

For a more cooling version of this cleansing dish, omit the garlic. Other vegetables, such as mushrooms and asparagus, could be added according to your tastes and the qualities you need. Serves 4.

> 6 *baby artichokes or the hearts of* 3 *large artichokes*
> *juice of* 1 *lemon*
> 225 *g/8 oz long-grain brown rice*
> 2 *garlic cloves, peeled and finely chopped (optional)*
> 1 *teaspoon salt*
> 25 *g/1 oz butter or 2 tablespoons olive oil*

Prepare the artichokes as described above, paring large artichokes right down so that only edible parts remain. Cut the artichoke hearts or baby artichokes into quarters or sixths. Sprinkle the cut surfaces with lemon juice, then put the artichokes into a heavy-based saucepan with the rice, the garlic if using, salt and 600 ml/1 pint water. Bring to the boil, then turn the heat right down, put a lid on the pan, and leave to cook very gently for 40–45 minutes. Gently stir in the butter or oil with a fork, fluffing the rice at the same time.

ASPARAGUS *Asparagus officinalis*

Cool to neutral, diuretic

The main benefit of asparagus is for KIDNEY PROBLEMS; it works as a diuretic, to eliminate fluid and increase urination.

Asparagus also has a mild tonic action on the whole system and a mild cleansing effect on the blood, so it can be helpful for SKIN PROBLEMS. It is thought to be effective against RHEUMATISM. And Dr Valnet considered asparagus to be mildly helpful for DIABETES and other imbalances of sugar metabolism. It is said to have a mild tonic action on the heart and lungs.

Note: Some authorities advise that asparagus should not be taken during the acute phases of an inflammatory disease, either of the kidneys or any other organ.

Preparing and Using: Asparagus should be washed, trimmed and then boiled until just tender: this can be anything from 2 to 15 minutes, depending on the thickness of the stalks. A good way to cook asparagus is flat, in a frying pan, with enough boiling water to cover it. Boil the asparagus until only just tender. Drain well (keep the water for stock), and serve with some olive oil or butter and a squeeze of lemon juice if you like. Some buttered brown rice goes well with this, to make a cleansing, light meal. Asparagus is also excellent served cold, as a salad, with olive oil and lemon juice.

ASPARAGUS SOUP

This soup is made from the trimmings of the asparagus. You could steam the tips and add them to the soup at the end to make it more luxurious, or serve them at another meal. Serves 4.

> *25 g/1 oz butter or 2 tablespoons olive oil*
> *1 small onion, peeled and chopped*
> *1 medium-sized potato, peeled and diced*
> *tough stalk ends and trimmings from 450 g/1 lb asparagus*
> *sea salt and freshly ground black pepper*
> *4 tablespoons single cream (optional)*

89

Heat the butter or oil in a large saucepan, then stir in the onion, potato and asparagus. Cover and cook over a gentle heat for 10 minutes, stirring from time to time. Add 1 litre/1¾ pints water, bring to the boil, then simmer for about 15 minutes, until the vegetables are cooked. Liquidise, and pass through a sieve if necessary to remove any stringy bits. Season to taste with salt and pepper, reheat, and add the cream if using.

ASPARAGUS WITH ORANGE AND ALMONDS

Serves 2.

> *225 g/8 oz asparagus*
> *1 unwaxed orange, well-scrubbed*
> *25 g/1 oz butter*
> *25 g/1 oz flaked almonds*

Trim the asparagus as necessary. Steam or cook as described above until just tender, then drain. Meanwhile, grate the rind from the orange, squeeze the juice and reserve. Melt the butter in a small saucepan and fry the almonds for 1−2 minutes until golden brown. Put the asparagus on a plate or plates, then add the orange rind and juice to the almonds in the pan, stir quickly and pour over the asparagus. Serve immediately.

AUBERGINE (EGG PLANT) *Solanum melongena*

Cooling

Aubergine has a mild therapeutic action in cooling an OVERHEATED LIVER and abdomen, and relieving DIGESTIVE CRAMP and hot, burning DIARRHOEA. It helps burning irritation and yellow GENITAL DISCHARGES, and is mildly diuretic. A recent report from China indicates that aubergine may help prevent the hardening of blood vessels and could be useful in the treatment of ATHEROSCLEROSIS.

Preparing and Using: The usual advice is first to slice the aubergine, then to sprinkle it with salt, and leave for 30 minutes to draw out the bitter juices. In practice, it is rare for aubergines to taste bitter, although this process does prevent the aubergine from absorbing too much fat. It's optional, however, if you are going to steam or bake it, as in the recipes below.

Aubergine can be fried in olive oil and served with lemon slices and a yogurt and herb or mayonnaise sauce; or cooked gently in olive oil with onions, garlic, tomatoes and other vegetables to make ratatouille and similar dishes. It can be baked whole, like a baked potato, then mashed or puréed with olive oil, lemon juice, seasoning and fresh herbs, to make a dip or salad dressing (perhaps with some tahini added). You may also enjoy it baked then stuffed, or steamed and marinated, as in the recipes below.

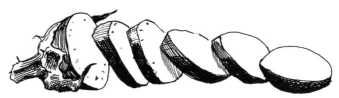

MARINATED AUBERGINE

In this simple dish the aubergine is warmed with the addition of ginger. For a more cooling dish, the ginger can be left out or replaced with chopped mint. Serve with cooked brown rice and stir-fried mixed vegetables. Serves 1–2.

> 1 *aubergine (about 350 g/12 oz)*
> *salt*
> For the marinade:
> 1 *tablespoon grated raw ginger*
> 1 *teaspoon sesame oil (optional)*
> 1 *teaspoon honey or Barbados sugar*
> 4 *tablespoons shoyu soy sauce*

Slice the aubergine into circles, then cut each into quarters. Put them in a colander, sprinkle with salt, place a weighted plate on top and leave for 30 minutes to draw out any bitter juices. Now rinse the aubergine under the cold tap, squeeze out as much water as possible, and steam for about 5 minutes, or until tender.

Meanwhile, mix together the ginger, sesame oil if using, honey or sugar, and soy sauce. Place the aubergine in a single layer in a shallow dish, and spoon the marinade over, making sure that all the aubergine pieces are coated. Leave for at least 1 hour – preferably longer – and spoon the marinade over the aubergine from time to time. Serve cold, or reheat gently in a covered dish over a pan of boiling water.

91

STUFFED AUBERGINE WITH HERBY TOPPING

Serves 2.

> 1 *large aubergine*
> 1 *onion, peeled and chopped*
> 2 *tablespoons olive oil*
> 1 *garlic clove, peeled and crushed*
> 100 *g/4 oz mushrooms, washed and sliced*
> 2 *tomatoes, skinned and chopped*
> *sea salt and freshly ground black pepper*
> 2 *tablespoons soft wholewheat breadcrumbs*
> 1 *tablespoon chopped fresh thyme*

Bake the aubergine whole in the oven at 200°C/400°F/Gas Mark 6 for about 30 minutes, until it feels tender. Allow to cool, then cut in half horizontally and scoop out the inside, keeping the skin intact. Fry the onion in 1 tablespoon oil for 5 minutes, then add the garlic and mushrooms, and fry for a further 5 minutes. Roughly chop the scooped-out aubergine flesh and add to the pan, together with the tomatoes. Stir until heated through, then remove from the heat and season with salt and pepper to taste.

Put the aubergine skins in a shallow casserole dish which will fit under the grill, then divide the mushroom mixture between them. Mix the breadcrumbs with the thyme and the remaining oil and sprinkle this on top of the stuffed aubergines. Place under a moderate grill for 5–10 minutes, or until the filling is hot and the topping is crisp and lightly browned. Alternatively, they can be baked at 200°C/400°F/Gas Mark 6 for about 20 minutes.

BEETROOT *Beta vulgaris*

Neutral to cooling, blood tonic

Beetroot has the ability to strengthen and cool the blood, promoting a clear and pink skin. It cools the digestive system, helping in burning, acidity, GASTRITIS and HAEMORRHOIDS (PILES). It can cool an OVERHEATED LIVER AND GALL BLADDER, signs of which are red eyes, 'BURSTING' HEADACHES, CONSTIPATION and anger. Beetroot also has a mildly tonic effect on the heart, like pomegranate.

Recent research in Europe, especially in Germany, has shown that taking at least 1 glass of raw beetroot juice each day can be helpful for CANCER. You can often buy the juice from healthfood shops. If you don't like the flavour, beetroot juice can be mixed with other fruit or vegetable juices such as orange, apple, carrot or celery. Beetroot can also be made into a soup or salad, or eaten hot with melted butter.

Preparing and Using: Although you can buy ready-cooked beetroot, this often has added vinegar or preservatives. It's really better to buy it raw and cook it yourself. To do this, cut off the leaves, if still attached, 10 cm/4 in above the beetroot and don't cut or peel the beetroot, as this encourages the colour to drain out.

Cover the beetroot with cold water, bring to the boil, then simmer, with a lid on the pan, for 1–3 hours, until tender. (A pressure cooker can speed this process up, of course.) Slip the skins off, then slice or cube the beetroot. When prepared like this, beetroot can be reheated with a little butter or olive oil and a squeeze of lemon juice. Cold, it's good mixed with sliced raw fennel, a few walnut pieces or chopped fresh herbs, or topped with a spoonful of soured cream or thick yogurt; some horseradish sauce stirred into the soured cream or yogurt makes a pleasantly pungent addition.

HEARTY BEETROOT SOUP

This is good for DIGESTIVE OR LIVER/GALL-BLADDER PROBLEMS when there is stagnation of energy shown as tiredness, coldness and depression. (It may help other stagnant energy problems, too.) Very healing to the digestive system, this nourishing soup is a meal in itself, although a little well-cooked brown rice and buckwheat could be served with it if you wish. Serves 3–4.

> 1 *tablespoon olive oil*
> 1 *onion, peeled and sliced*
> 2 *garlic cloves, peeled and crushed*
> 2 *carrots, scrubbed and chopped*
> 225 *g/8 oz beetroot, peeled and diced*
> 225 *g/8 oz cabbage, roughly chopped*
> 225 *g/8 oz potato, peeled and diced*
> *sea salt*

Heat the oil in a large saucepan, then put in the onion, garlic and all the vegetables. Stir, then cover and cook gently for 10 minutes. Add 600 ml/1 pint water, bring to the boil, then simmer for a further 20–30 minutes, or until all the vegetables are tender. Remove a ladleful of the soup and liquidise until smooth; return this to the pan to thicken the soup. Season to taste with salt, and reheat. For an extra-luxurious version, serve with a spoonful of soured cream on each portion and a good sprinkling of chopped dill or chives.

C A B B A G E *Brassica oleracea*

Cool, anti-inflammatory

This vegetable has been cultivated in the West for over 4000 years and many European naturopaths consider it to be one of the greatest healers of the vegetable kingdom. The great French natural doctor, Dr Valnet, calls cabbage 'the medicine of the poor'.

Cabbage is useful both externally and internally. Dr Valnet cites many cases in which the application of slightly crushed cabbage leaves to gangrenous wounds brought healing, in some instances even avoiding the need for surgery or amputation. You can apply cabbage leaves externally to any part of the body which is inflamed, including RHEU-MATIC JOINTS and GANGRENE. Bind the leaves firmly in position and leave them overnight, using fresh leaves for each application. The leaves will draw off the toxins, cooling and healing the painful area. Many other French doctors, including Dr Blanc and Dr Leclerc, vouch for this remedy, which was also used in ancient times by Greek and Roman physicians such as Galen, Hippocrates and Pliny.

Cabbage cools the digestive system, and is therefore effective for INDIGESTION where there is not only swelling and flatulence but also acidity, burning and inflammation, as in GASTRITIS and ULCERS. The ability of cabbage to heal digestive ulcers has been known for centuries. In 1557 a Dutchman, Dr Dodens, wrote: 'the juice of cabbage soothes the abdomen and relieves constipation, cleans and heals old ulcers both internal and external. Mixed with honey, makes a syrup that cures hoarseness and cough.' Recently researchers have found in cabbage vitamin U, a substance which accounts for this healing property. It continues to be helpful for intestinal disorders such as CONSTIPATION, ULCERATIVE COLITIS and IRRITABLE BOWEL SYNDROME.

The most effective way to take cabbage for these conditions is in the form of juice (see below). Cabbage juice also loosens mucus in the respiratory system, thus making it easier for expectorants to expel it. This treatment is also helpful for DRY COUGHS and WEAK LUNGS.

Juice or soup made from cabbage is considered useful for INFLAMMA-TIONS OF THE BLADDER when there may be burning, discharges and

94

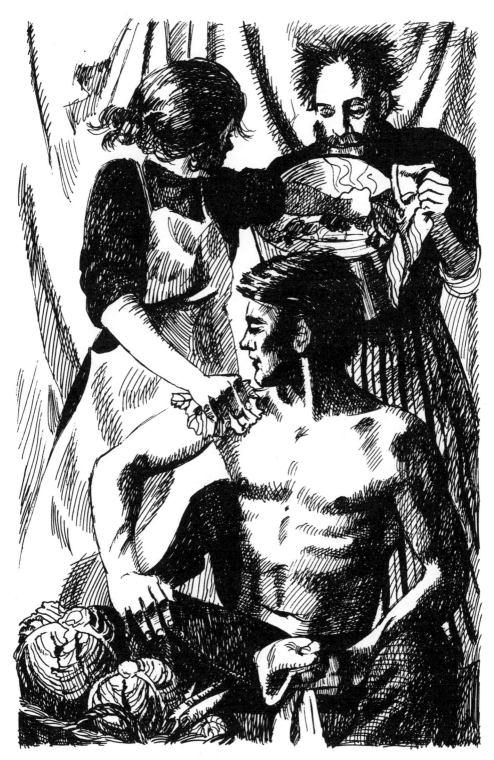

A cabbage-leaf poultice

difficulties in urination. In men, these remedies can soothe an INFLAMED PROSTATE.

Cabbage juice can be extracted either with a juicer, or by liquidising the cabbage and then pressing it through a sieve or squeezing it in muslin. As a treatment, the juice can be taken on its own or diluted with water – look under specific illnesses for detailed instructions. For a refreshing drink which is also cleansing and soothing, mix a small quantity of cabbage juice with other juices such as apple, carrot and celery.

Preparing and Using: Choose a firm, hearty cabbage such as Primo rather than white 'salad cabbage', and try different types of *Brassica* such as spring greens, Brussels sprouts and broccoli, all of which share the qualities described. (Red cabbage has much the same properties as white or green, except that it is slightly less anti-inflammatory and rather more strengthening to the blood.) Shred the cabbage finely and mix with lemon juice and olive oil, mayonnaise, yogurt or soured cream and fresh herbs or spices – caraway seeds are especially good – for cabbage salads.

The secret of cooked cabbage is to cook it quickly and lightly, until only just tender, in the minimum of water. Shred the cabbage well, then put it into a small quantity of boiling water – not more than a scant 1 cm/ ½ in – and put a lid on the pan. The cabbage will half-boil, half-steam in the water and will take 4–7 minutes, until it is just tender and still bright green. When you get used to this method you will probably find that you use even less water – just enough to prevent the cabbage from sticking to the bottom of the pan.

Drain the cabbage (keeping the water for stock) and add a little butter or oil, a small amount of sea salt and any spices or chopped herbs that you like, or which have the properties you need. For a simple, cleansing meal, serve the cabbage with a cooked grain such as brown rice.

CABBAGE SALAD FOR A HANGOVER

This may not be exactly what you fancy when you wake up with a hangover, but it does work for some people. If you can't face a salad, try the other suggestions on page 216. Serves 1.

> 175 g/6 oz white cabbage
> a sweet eating apple, quartered and cored (optional)
> juice of ½–1 lemon
> sea salt

Grate or finely chop the cabbage and apple, preferably in a food-processor, reducing them to an almost purée-like consistency. Add the lemon juice and a little salt to taste.

CABBAGE AND POTATO SOUP WITH THYME AND FENNEL

This is a wonderfully warming and soothing soup for COUGHS, CATARRH and BRONCHITIS. You can make it thick and chunky or add more liquid and whizz it to a smooth, creamy consistency. If you like a richer soup, a little cream can be added at the end. Serves 4.

15 g/½ oz butter
1 small cabbage, trimmed and shredded
1 large potato, peeled and diced
½ teaspoon fennel seeds
½ teaspoon thyme
sea salt and freshly ground black pepper

Melt the butter in a large saucepan and stir in the cabbage, potato, fennel seeds and thyme. Then cover and cook without browning for 10 minutes, stirring from time to time. Add 1 litre/1¾ pints water, cover the pan and leave the soup to simmer for about 20 minutes, until the potatoes are tender. Liquidise all or some of the soup, or leave it as it is; season with a little salt and pepper to taste.

CABBAGE, PUMPKIN, FENNEL AND CARROT SOUP WITH ANISEED

A wonderfully soothing soup for COLITIS and ULCERS, this also helps CONSTIPATION. Serves 4.

25 g/1 oz butter or 2 tablespoons olive oil
225 g/8 oz cabbage, shredded
225 g/8 oz pumpkin (weighed after removing skin and seeds)
225 g/8 oz fennel, sliced
225 g/8 oz carrots, scraped and diced
1 teaspoon aniseed
sea salt

Heat the butter or oil in a large saucepan, then stir in the cabbage, pumpkin, fennel, carrots and aniseed. Cover and cook gently for

97

10 minutes, stirring from time to time. Add 1 litre/1¾ pints water, bring to the boil, then simmer gently for a further 15 minutes or so until the vegetables are tender. Season lightly with salt. This soup can be served as it is, with chunky pieces of vegetable; or it can be partially liquidised, with some chunks of vegetable in a creamy base; or wholly liquidised to a creamy consistency.

BUBBLE AND SQUEAK

A traditional British economy dish which is also a tasty way to enjoy the healing properties of cabbage. Herbs and spices can be added according to your needs. Serves 2.

> 450 g/1 lb potatoes, peeled and cut into even-sized chunks
> 450 g/1 lb cabbage, shredded
> 1 teaspoon fennel or caraway seeds (optional)
> lemon juice
> sea salt
> 2 tablespoons olive oil

Put the potatoes in enough water to cover and boil for about 20 minutes until tender. Mash roughly. Meanwhile, cook the cabbage in the minimum of boiling water – 1 cm/½ in or less – for about 5 minutes, until just tender, then drain. Mix together the cabbage and potatoes, add the fennel or caraway seeds if using, and lemon juice and salt to taste. Heat the oil in a frying pan, preferably non-stick, then put in the cabbage and potato mixture and press down to make a flat 'cake'. Fry until crisp and brown, then turn over (you may need to cut the 'cake' into quarters with a fish slice or spatula in order to do this) and fry the other side.

SPICED CABBAGE AND CARROTS

This is soothing and helpful for the stomach and digestion. Serve it with brown rice, perhaps some SPICY LENTIL DAL (page 144) and some chopped cucumber mixed with goat's milk yogurt, for a complete meal. Other spices can be used to help specific conditions; add a teaspoonful of grated fresh ginger, for instance, for its warming qualities, if appropriate. Serves 2.

> 2 tablespoons olive oil
> 1 teaspoon cumin seeds

1 teaspoon coriander seeds, crushed
350 g/12 oz cabbage, shredded
350 g/12 oz carrots, scraped and coarsely grated
lemon juice
sea salt
chopped fresh coriander, if available

Heat the oil in a large saucepan; put in the cumin and coriander seeds and stir for a few seconds. Then add the cabbage and carrots, stirring well. Add 2 tablespoons water, stir again, then turn down the heat, cover and cook for about 5 minutes, or until the vegetables are tender. Add a little lemon juice and salt to taste, sprinkle with chopped fresh coriander if available, and serve.

STIR-FRIED VEGETABLES WITH FRESH GINGER

A variation of the previous recipe, this time with a Chinese influence. This is good with plain boiled brown rice and extra soy sauce to sprinkle over. Serves 2.

2 tablespoons olive oil
1 teaspoon grated ginger
225 g/8 oz cabbage, shredded
100 g/4 oz carrots, scrubbed and sliced diagonally
175 g/6 oz courgettes, sliced thinly, diagonally
175 g/6 oz baby sweetcorn
100 g/4 oz mangetouts
2 tablespoons soy sauce
sea salt

Heat the oil in a large pan or wok, put in the ginger, cabbage and carrots and stir well. Cover and cook over a low heat for 5 minutes, then add the courgettes and cook for a further 4–5 minutes. Now put in the sweetcorn and mangetouts, and stir-fry for another 1–2 minutes. Add the soy sauce and a little salt if necessary, and serve at once.

CARROTS *Daucus carota*

Neutral, tonic, anti-inflammatory

The therapeutic qualities of carrots have been noted throughout the ages; these have perhaps been explained in part by the discovery in more modern times of their high content of carotene, precursor to vitamin A.

Carrots soothe the inflamed mucus membranes which underlie DRY COUGHS, SORE THROATS, GASTRITIS, ULCERS and similar conditions. They also strengthen resistance to COLDS AND FLU, a quality which is reinforced by combining carrot with some lemon or lime juice.

The action of carrots on the intestines is pronounced. They have an anti-inflammatory action, helping to heal conditions such as ULCERATIVE COLITIS and IRRITABLE BOWEL SYNDROME. They also have a regulatory effect on the bowel, improving CONSTIPATION but at the same time reducing DIARRHOEA.

A SCALY, DRY SKIN is moistened by eating carrots, and HOT RHEUMATISM is eased. Carrots protect and strengthen eyesight, particularly when eaten raw or in the form of juice.

Preparing and Using: One of the most useful vegetables, carrots are good raw in salads, cooked, or in the form of juice. Scrape the carrots as thinly as possible, or simply scrub them if they're young and tender; then grate, slice or dice as required. They are best cooked in a steamer over boiling water until just tender: 5–15 minutes, depending on the size. Alternatively, you could toss them in a little melted butter or oil, put a lid on the pan and cook for about 5 minutes. Then add just enough water to stop the carrots sticking to the pan, cover again and cook for a further 5–15 minutes, until just tender. Dried herbs and spices such as aniseed, cumin, caraway and coriander can be added during the cooking time; or fresh herbs such as chopped parsley can be sprinkled on top just before serving.

To improve the skin, mix equal quantities of carrot juice (if you haven't got a juicer, make this in the same way as cabbage juice, page 96) and fresh apricot juice. Apricot nectar (available from some supermarkets) can be used, but check the ingredients list to make sure that the juice is pure, with no sugar or other additives.

STIR-FRIED CARROT, CABBAGE, LEEKS AND
FENNEL WITH ORANGE

This delicious combination of vegetables is good for CONSTIPATION. It makes a complete light meal as it is, although you could serve it with some cooked brown rice or another grain, or some good bread. Serves 2.

2 large bulbs of fennel
225 g/8 oz carrots
225 g/8 oz cabbage
225 g/8 oz leeks
2–4 tablespoons olive oil
grated rind of 1 unwaxed orange
juice of 1 lemon
sea salt

Trim and slice the fennel; scrape the carrots, then grate them coarsely or slice them thinly, perhaps into matchsticks. Shred the cabbage; trim the roots and any tough green leaves off the leeks, slit them up the side if necessary to wash them thoroughly, then slice thinly. Heat 2 tablespoons olive oil in a large pan or wok. Put in the vegetables and stir-fry for 1–2 minutes. When they are all coated with the oil, cover, turn the heat down, and leave to cook gently for 5–10 minutes, until the vegetables are tender. Add the orange rind, lemon juice and sea salt to taste, and another 1–2 tablespoons olive oil if you wish. Serve immediately.

CARROT AND NUTMEG SAUCE

This gentle, soothing mixture goes well with many other vegetables. Try serving it with steamed courgettes or cabbage, and brown rice, or with BIRCHER POTATOES (page 123). With more water added, it becomes a carrot soup (see also the recipe for CABBAGE, PUMPKIN, FENNEL AND CARROT SOUP WITH ANISEED, page 97). Serves 2–4.

25 g/1 oz butter
1 onion, peeled and chopped
750 g/1½ lb carrots, scrubbed and sliced
sea salt
honey
grated nutmeg

Melt the butter in a large saucepan. Add the onion and carrots, cover and sauté gently for 10 minutes: don't let them burn. Now add 150 ml/5 fl oz water, bring to the boil, cover again and simmer for a further 10 minutes, until the carrots are tender. Liquidise to a smooth purée, adding more water if you want a thinner consistency. Season with salt, a dash of honey and a little grated nutmeg.

101

CARROT, COURGETTE, THYME AND GINGER SOUP

This is a light but warming soup and it's pretty to look at, orange flecked with shades of green. Serves 4.

> *350 g/12 oz carrots, scraped and sliced*
> *1 teaspoon thyme*
> *1–2 teaspoons grated fresh ginger*
> *125 g/4 oz courgettes, coarsely grated*
> *sea salt and freshly ground black pepper*

Put the carrots in a saucepan with the thyme, ginger and 1 litre/1¾ pints water. Bring to the boil, then cover and simmer for about 15 minutes, until the carrots are tender. Liquidise until smooth, return to the saucepan and add the grated courgettes. Simmer for a further 3–5 minutes, or until the courgettes are just tender. Season with salt and pepper to taste. Add a little butter before serving if you like.

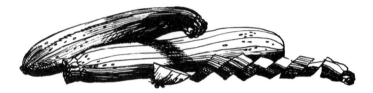

CELERY *Apium graveolens*

Cooling, diuretic, tonic, beneficial for the nerves

Celery is particularly helpful for KIDNEY PROBLEMS. Like artichokes and asparagus, it cleanses and strengthens these organs. As an effective diuretic, it eliminates OEDEMA (FLUID RETENTION). It cools and improves digestion, and is also helpful in RHEUMATISM, especially when the joints look red and inflamed.

During times of STRESS and overwork, celery is said to strengthen the nervous system whilst at the same time calming it and promoting relaxation and sleep. It is also recommended for HYPERTENSION (HIGH BLOOD PRESSURE).

Preparing and Using: Celery is good raw, in salads and with dips; cooked as a vegetable, or in soups and stews; and in the form of juice. Try mixing celery juice with equal parts of carrot juice and apple juice for a particularly refreshing drink.

102

BUTTERED CELERY

Serves 4–6.

> *4 celery hearts or 2 large heads of celery*
> *25 g/1 oz butter*
> *sea salt and freshly ground black pepper*

Wash the celery under the cold tap without taking the heads apart, then cut the hearts downwards into halves or quarters. If you're using 2 large heads, cut off the sticks about 15 cm/6 in above the base, then cut the hearts into quarters. Cut the remaining pieces of celery into 5 cm/2 in pieces. Put all the celery in a large saucepan, add enough cold water to come halfway up the celery, add a little salt, then cover, bring to the boil, and simmer for about 20 minutes, or 7 minutes in a pressure-cooker, until the celery is tender. Drain the water from the celery (keeping it for stock) and add the butter to the pan. Cover and let the celery cook for a further 10 minutes, or until very tender and buttery. Season to taste with salt and pepper.

Celery cooked this way can be put into a flameproof dish, sprinkled with Parmesan cheese (if your diet allows this) and browned for 1–2 minutes under a hot grill; or it can be finished with SAVOURY CRUMBLE TOPPING (page 161) and baked in the oven, for a more substantial dish.

CELERY AND OATMEAL BROTH WITH BASIL AND MARJORAM

A soothing, creamy soup, to relax the nervous system and promote sound sleep. You could use the leftover celery heart to make the salad which follows this recipe. Serves 4.

> *outside sticks from 1 head of celery*
> *50 g/2 oz rolled oats*
> *½ teaspoon dried basil*
> *½ teaspoon dried marjoram*
> *25 g/1 oz butter (optional)*
> *sea salt*
> *chopped fresh basil*

Wash and chop the celery, then put it into a large saucepan with 1 litre/ 1¾ pints water, the oats, dried basil and marjoram. Half cover, bring to the boil, then simmer gently for about 30 minutes, or until the celery is tender. Liquidise with the butter, if using. Season to taste with a little salt. Reheat gently, and serve with some fresh basil chopped over the top.

CELERY, CARROT AND APPLE SALAD

This is a delicious salad, cooling and soothing for an OVERHEATED DIGESTION. Serves 2.

>*2 large carrots, scraped and grated*
>*2 apples, grated*
>*1 celery heart, sliced*
>*juice of 1 lemon*
>*a little sea salt (optional)*
>*chopped fresh mint*

Mix all the ingredients together and serve.

CHICORY (WILD) *Cichorium intybus*

Cool, moist, cleansing

The type of chicory referred to here is not the yellow-green salad vegetable, but a wild plant with thin, dark green leaves, much used in Europe. As with dandelion, both the leaves and the root of this plant are useful. They have a strong effect on the digestive system, being especially beneficial for a congested OVERHEATED LIVER, but also improving the action of the intestines. They can be of great help in relieving CONSTIPATION. Chicory cleanses the blood and is useful in treating red and INFLAMED SKIN CONDITIONS; it is also a diuretic. Dr Valnet recommends chicory for people with DIABETES, and HYPOGLYCAEMIA.

Chicory root is sold in healthfood shops as a coffee substitute; it can also be bought mixed with coffee, a combination which is particularly popular in France.

Preparing and Using: These long green leaves are not often available in England although they can be grown if you have a garden. To cook them, steam the leaves lightly, then pan-fry them briefly with a whole clove of garlic and a little oil. If you want to make them more warming in their action, add half a green or red chilli to the mixture (remove the garlic and chillies, if used, before serving). For a mixture which is excellent for CONSTIPATION, and also a delicious dish in its own right, steam equal quantities of chicory, leeks, fennel, artichoke hearts, onions and mooli (or white radish). Then, before serving, toss them in virgin olive oil and add a good quantity of raw mooli, either finely chopped or grated. If you can't get chicory, use spinach or chard instead.

COURGETTE *Cucurbita pepo*

Cooling, anti-inflammatory, anti-spasmodic

The main action of courgettes is to cool and soothe the digestive system. They are valuable for hot types of INDIGESTION, ULCERS, GASTRITIS and COLITIS, soothing the digestive lining, calming spasms and alleviating soreness. They have a mildly calming effect on a tense digestion due to NERVOUS STRESS.

Marrow, which is really a large courgette, has similar properties.

Preparing and Using: Tender courgettes can be sliced thinly or grated and served raw in salads or with dips. Or they can be cooked lightly in water or butter. One of the nicest ways is to steam or boil them until almost tender, then toss them in butter and add some chopped fresh herbs, such as marjoram, tarragon or thyme.

Marrow is best cooked gently in a little butter or olive oil and water. You'll need to peel, then slice or dice the marrow, removing the seeds only if they're tough. Heat 15 g/½ oz butter or 1 tablespoon oil in a heavy-based saucepan and put in the marrow. Stir for a few seconds to ensure that all the pieces get coated with the butter or oil, then add 4 tablespoons water. Turn the heat down, cover, and leave to cook very gently for about 10 minutes, or until the marrow is tender and looks translucent. Herbs and spices can be added as required; fennel seeds and aniseed go particularly well with cooked marrow.

COURGETTE, POTATO AND ONION SOUP

The soothing, diuretic properties of this soup make it particularly helpful for KIDNEY AND BLADDER INFLAMMATIONS. Serves 4.

> 1 *large potato, peeled and diced*
> 1 *large onion, peeled and sliced*
> 450 *g/1 lb courgettes, sliced*
> *sea salt and freshly ground black pepper*
> *grated nutmeg (optional)*
> 25 *g/1 oz butter (optional)*

105

Put the potato and onion in a large saucepan with 1 litre/1¾ pints water, and simmer for 15 minutes. Add the courgettes, cover and continue to cook for a further 5 minutes, until the vegetables are tender. Season with salt and pepper, and add the grated nutmeg and butter if using. This soup can be served as it is, with chunky pieces of vegetable, or it can be wholly or partially liquidised, as you wish.

COURGETTES WITH WALNUT STUFFING

This is good served with CARROT AND NUTMEG SAUCE (page 101) and sweetcorn or cooked brown rice. Serves 2.

> 2 × 175 g/6 oz courgettes
> 1 quantity Walnut Stuffing (page 175)

Preheat the oven to 200°C/400°F/Gas Mark 6. Cut the stalks off the courgettes and halve them lengthwise. Then use a teaspoon to scoop out the seeds, leaving a cavity for the stuffing. Parboil the courgettes for 4 minutes, then drain and blot dry with kitchen paper.

Now make the walnut stuffing, frying the scooped-out courgette with the onion as described. Pack the stuffing into the courgette cavities, piling it up well. Put the stuffed courgette halves into a shallow oven-proof dish and bake, uncovered, for 15–20 minutes, or until the stuffing is lightly browned and the courgettes tender.

COURGETTES WITH CORIANDER

Serve this with new or mashed potato for a particularly soothing combination of vegetables; it's also good with brown rice. Or you could add a STUFFED AUBERGINE (page 92) for ratatouille vegetables with a difference. Serves 2 as a main dish.

> 2 peppers (red, green or yellow)
> 1 tablespoon olive oil
> 1 onion, peeled and sliced
> 1 garlic clove, peeled and crushed
> 2 teaspoons coriander seeds, roughly crushed
> 2 courgettes, trimmed and diced
> 3 tomatoes, skinned and chopped
> sea salt and freshly ground black pepper

First prepare the peppers by cutting them into quarters and removing

106

the seeds. Place them, shiny side up, under quite a fierce grill for a few minutes until the skins blister, char slightly and loosen. Remove from the grill, cover to let the steam further loosen the skins, then remove the skins with a sharp knife and cut the peppers into strips. Warm the oil in a saucepan and add the onion, garlic and peppers. Fry for 4–5 minutes, then add the coriander seeds, courgettes and tomatoes. Stir, then cook for about 20 minutes, or until the vegetables are tender. Season to taste with salt and pepper. This is good either hot or cold.

CUCUMBER *Cucurbita citrullus*

Cooling, cleansing, diuretic

Cucumber cools the stomach and digestion and is thus beneficial eaten before or after a hot and spicy meal as the Indians do, with their refreshing raitas of cucumber, yogurt and mint.

Hot and dry RESPIRATORY CONDITIONS are also eased by cucumber, as is hot and intoxicated blood creating SKIN INFLAMMATION. For this condition, slices of cucumber can also be applied externally as a poultice, or the cucumber can be grated so that it is semi-liquid, and used to massage the affected area.

Preparing and Using: Cucumber is usually used raw, peeled or unpeeled, sliced or chopped. It is, however, also delicious cooked. Peel the cucumber and cut into 1 cm/½ in slices. Melt 25 g/1 oz butter in a heavy-based saucepan and put in the cucumber, with 1 teaspoon fennel seeds or a bay leaf or any other spices you fancy. Cover and leave to cook gently for about 10 minutes, stirring from time to time, until the cucumber is very tender and looks translucent. Season to taste with sea salt and freshly ground black pepper.

CUCUMBER RAITA WITH FRESH MINT

This salad can be served as a cooling accompaniment to spicy dishes; it is also good spooned over lettuce hearts for a refreshing summer salad, or served as a dip. It's best made just before you want to eat it, to avoid the cucumber juices making it too watery. Serves 1–4.

> *½ cucumber*
> *150 g/5 oz thick Greek yogurt*
> *several sprigs of fresh mint, chopped*
> *sea salt*

Peel the cucumber and cut into small dice. Mix with the yogurt, mint and salt to taste. Serve immediately.

COOLING SUMMER SALAD

This is a cooling and detoxifying salad. Serves 1.

> ¼ *hearty lettuce, torn or shredded*
> ¼ *cucumber, sliced thinly*
> ½ *firm beefsteak tomato, sliced*
> *a small handful of watercress*
> *virgin olive oil*
> *sea salt*
> *lemon juice*

Arrange the lettuce, cucumber, tomato and watercress on a plate or put them in a small salad bowl. Sprinkle over a little olive oil, salt to taste and a squeeze of lemon juice just before serving.

DANDELION *Taraxacum officinale*

Cooling, cleansing, tonic

Dandelion has many beneficial properties and its importance is noted in natural healing traditions all over the world. Both the leaves and the root can be used, the root as a decoction and the leaves in salads, soups or tea. They improve the digestion and reduce inflammation in the digestive tract, helping ULCERS, COLITIS, DIVERTICULITIS and similar conditions; they cleanse and cool the blood, thus helping to soothe SKIN INFLAMMATIONS; they reduce SWELLINGS IN THE SPLEEN, and they cleanse the lymphatic system and eliminate NODULES. Dandelion leaves and root also increase the flow of milk in nursing mothers.

French herbalists say that dandelions clear the liver and wash the kidneys. They are certainly valuable for clearing and regenerating a congested OVERHEATED LIVER, and they have a similar effect on CONGESTED KIDNEYS. Dandelion, particularly the root, is a powerful diuretic, good for eliminating OEDEMA (FLUID RETENTION) and helpful for WEIGHT LOSS. While chemical diuretics can inflame the kidneys and cause the body to lose potassium and other minerals, dandelions contain anti-inflammatory substances and are rich in minerals, such as potassium. Dandelion leaves are also very rich in vitamin A.

Preparing and Using: Pick tender leaves from an unpolluted place. The leaves can be chopped and made into tea or they can be added to salads. They have a pleasantly bitter taste which is particularly good in a green salad. Dandelion root can be scrubbed, steamed and eaten as a vegetable, or the liquid can be drunk as a decoction.

You can also take dandelion root in the form of a coffee substitute. For this the roots need to be scrubbed, roasted until dry and brown, and then ground. It takes a large quantity of dandelion root to produce a small amount of coffee, so you may find it easier to buy dandelion coffee in healthfood shops. Pure dandelion coffee is the best; it is made by simmering the pieces in water for 5–10 minutes, or the root can be ground and used in a filter or cafetière in the same way as ordinary coffee.

DANDELION LEAF SALAD WITH HOT GARLIC CROÛTONS

Serves 4.

> 1 *lettuce*
> *a handful of tender dandelion leaves, well-washed*
> 3 *tablespoons olive oil*
> *juice of ½ lemon*
> *sea salt*
> For the garlic croûtons:
> *oil for frying*
> 4 *slices wholewheat bread, crusts removed and bread cut into*
> *5 mm/¼ in cubes*
> 2 *garlic cloves, peeled and crushed*

Tear or shred the lettuce and dandelion leaves and put them into a bowl or on to a serving plate. In a small bowl, mix the oil, lemon juice and a little salt.

Just before serving, make the croûtons. Cover the base of a frying pan generously with oil and heat. Then add the cubes of bread and the garlic and fry over a moderate heat, stirring constantly, until the croûtons are golden brown all over. Drain on crumpled kitchen paper.

Give the dressing a quick stir, then pour it over the salad, mix quickly, add the croûtons and serve immediately.

FENNEL *Foeniculum vulgare*

Anti-inflammatory, laxative

Fennel bulb has similar qualities to those described for fennel seed (page 55) except that the bulb is more cooling and anti-inflammatory. The main action of fennel is on the digestion, where it acts as a laxative, easing CONSTIPATION and helping to soothe inflammation.

Preparing and Using: With its fresh, aniseed flavour, and crisp yet tender texture, fennel is good either raw or cooked, and it makes a delicate and delicious soup. Trim off the stalk ends, base and any tough outer leaves, then slice, keeping any green leafy fronds for garnish. Fennel is good prepared in the ways described below, and the recipe for BUTTERED CELERY (page 103) also works very well with fennel.

FENNEL SOUP

An excellent soup for the digestive system and, because of its diuretic action, helpful for WEIGHT LOSS. You can make this soup without the preliminary sautéeing if you prefer; in this case, just simmer the chopped fennel in the water until tender. Serves 4.

> *2 large bulbs of fennel*
> *1 tablespoon olive oil*
> *sea salt and freshly ground black pepper*

Wash and chop the fennel, reserving any tender feathery leaves for garnish. Heat the oil in a large saucepan and sauté the fennel gently for 5–10 minutes, without browning. Add 1 litre/1¾ pints water, bring to the boil and simmer gently for 15–20 minutes, until the fennel is tender. Liquidise, then season to taste with salt and pepper, sprinkle over the reserved fennel leaves and serve.

FENNEL AND LETTUCE SALAD

This is a good salad to soothe an OVERHEATED DIGESTION, and helpful for CONSTIPATION. Serves 2.

> *1 bulb of fennel*
> *1 hearty lettuce (little gem type)*

110

a few black olives (optional)
virgin olive oil
juice of ½ lemon

Cut any tough stalk ends or leaves from the fennel, then slice it downwards into eighths or even thinner slices. Slice the lettuce heart in the same way. Arrange the slices on a serving plate, and scatter over the olives, if using. Just before serving, sprinkle with olive oil and pour the lemon juice on top.

FENNEL AND TOMATO VINAIGRETTE
WITH BLACK OLIVES

A refreshing and cooling mixture. Serves 1–2.

1 bulb of fennel
2–3 tomatoes
2–3 black olives
juice of ½ lemon
1–2 tablespoons olive oil
sea salt

Slice the fennel thinly and chop any tender green leaves. Slice the tomatoes. Put the fennel, tomatoes and olives into a shallow dish and sprinkle with the lemon juice, oil and a little salt. This salad improves if the flavours are allowed to blend for a while before eating. If you do not want to eat the fennel raw, it can be steamed lightly, then cooled, before using.

FENNEL WITH ORANGES AND BLACK OLIVES

Serves 2.

1 large bulb of fennel
2 oranges
6–8 black olives
a little virgin olive oil (optional)

Slice the fennel thinly and chop any tender green leaves. Cut the peel and pith from the oranges, then slice the oranges thinly. Mix together the fennel, oranges and black olives, sprinkle with a little olive oil if using, and serve.

111

FENNEL BULB WITH FENNEL SEEDS

This, and the next recipe, are delicious ways to eat health-giving fennel. They go well with many main dishes; served with brown rice and another dish, such as STIR-FRIED TOFU WITH CARROTS AND ONIONS (page 150), either of these recipes would make a complete meal. Or you could sprinkle a little grated Parmesan cheese on top of the fennel, and brown it under the grill, for a more substantial dish which could be served as a light main course, with another vegetable, such as spinach. Serves 2–3.

> 4 *medium-sized bulbs of fennel*
> 1 *tablespoon olive oil*
> 1 *teaspoon fennel seeds*
> *sea salt and freshly ground black pepper*

Wash and trim the fennel, keeping any tender leaves. Slice the fennel in half and then downwards into fairly chunky segments. Heat the oil in a frying pan, add the fennel, any pieces of leaf, and the fennel seeds. Stir-fry for a few minutes, then cover the frying pan. Let the fennel continue to cook, stirring from time to time, for 15–20 minutes, or until tender and slightly browned in places. Season to taste with salt and pepper.

FENNEL À LA GRECQUE

Serves 1–2.

> 1 *bulb of fennel*
> 2 *tablespoons olive oil*
> 1 *onion, peeled and chopped*
> 1 *garlic clove, peeled and crushed*
> 2 *teaspoons coriander seeds*
> 1 *tomato, skinned and chopped (optional)*
> *juice of ½ lemon*
> *sea salt*
> *freshly ground black pepper (optional)*
> *a dash of honey (optional)*

Wash and trim the fennel, keeping any tender leafy bits for garnish. Slice the fennel in half and then downwards into fairly thin segments. Boil or steam the fennel for about 5 minutes, until it begins to get tender, then drain well. Heat the oil in a frying pan and fry the onion for 5 minutes, then add the garlic and fennel. Crush the coriander seeds roughly, using a pestle and mortar or the back of a wooden spoon on a board. Add these to the fennel, together with the tomato if using, and the lemon juice. Stir, then cover and leave to cook for 15–20 minutes, or until the fennel is very tender. Season with salt, pepper if appropriate for your diet, and a dash of honey if needed. Serve warm or cold, with any reserved leafy pieces chopped over the top.

LEEK *Allium porrum*

Hot, expectorant

The main action of leeks is on the respiratory system, where they can first loosen the phlegm and then expectorate it. Leeks have antiseptic properties which help to clear the bacteria which can accumulate when there is EXCESSIVE PHLEGM. This antiseptic quality means that leeks also cleanse the whole of the digestive system, and they are a particularly good food to take for a SLOW DIGESTION. They are thought to stimulate intestinal peristalsis and they have a laxative action which is helpful for CONSTIPATION.

Leeks are a diuretic, increasing the urine flow and mildly cleansing the kidneys and bladder. Because of this action, leeks can assist WEIGHT LOSS, particularly in the form of a soup (see recipe below). For this purpose, they can also be combined with the other diuretic vegetables, fennel, asparagus and artichokes.

During the winter months leeks can be beneficial for COLD RHEUMATISM – the type with swelling joints and cramping pains, which is worse during cold weather – and for this they can be taken regularly, perhaps combined with thyme, ginger or oregano (see recipes below).

Leeks have a mildly cleansing effect on the blood and so can also improve SKIN PROBLEMS.

Preparing and Using: Trimmed, well-washed leeks can be cooked whole or sliced, either in a steamer or in 1 cm/½ in boiling water until just tender: 1–2 minutes for shredded leeks, 8–15 minutes for whole ones. Leeks cooked like this can be served with a little oil or melted butter and fresh or dried herbs, or spices, chosen for the particular healing properties you need.

LEEK AND GINGER SOUP

A warming soup, helpful for COUGHS, COLDS, SORE THROATS, and congestion in the nose or sinuses. As a variation, the leeks can simply be boiled in the water (without preliminary sautéeing) and liquidised to a cream when tender. If you want to make this creamy soup more substantial, a potato can be cooked with the leeks and you can adjust the consistency by adding more water after liquidising if necessary. Serves 4.

> *3 leeks*
> *1 tablespoon olive oil*
> *1 tablespoon grated fresh ginger*
> *sea salt and freshly ground black pepper*

Trim the roots and tough green leaves off the leeks, wash them thoroughly and slice thinly. Heat the oil in a large saucepan and sauté the leeks gently for 5–10 minutes, without browning. Add the ginger, stir, then add 1 litre/1¾ pints water. Cover, bring the soup to the boil and simmer gently for 15–20 minutes, until the leeks are tender. Season to taste with salt and pepper.

LEEK AND FENNEL SOUP

To help WEIGHT LOSS, this soup can be served as it is, with chunky pieces of vegetable, or liquidised to a smooth cream. Serves 4.

> *1 tablespoon olive oil*
> *2 leeks, washed and sliced*
> *1 large bulb of fennel, washed and chopped*
> *1 teaspoon fennel seeds*
> *sea salt and freshly ground black pepper*

Heat the oil in a large saucepan and sauté the leeks, fennel and fennel seeds gently for 5–10 minutes, without browning. Add 1 litre/1¾ pints water. Cover, bring the soup to the boil and simmer gently for 15–20 minutes, until the vegetables are tender. Season to taste with salt and pepper.

LEEKS WITH LEMON VINAIGRETTE

For a change, cooked leeks are good served cold, with a tangy lemon vinaigrette. This is nice as a first course, or, with one or two raw vegetables, such as grated carrot and some shredded lettuce, as part of a salad meal. Serves 2.

6 *thin leeks*
1 *unwaxed lemon, well-scrubbed*
4 *tablespoons olive oil*
sea salt
chopped fresh parsley

Trim the leeks, then slit them down the side and rinse under the cold tap to clean them. Cook the leeks in boiling water to cover until they are very tender, then drain well. (The cooking water makes good stock for soups.) Lay the leeks in a dish in a single layer. Grate or pare off thin threads of rind from the lemon and add these to the leeks. Squeeze the juice from the lemon; pour this over the leeks, then pour the oil evenly on top. Sprinkle with a little salt and leave to cool and marinate, turning the leeks over once or twice and spooning the liquid over them. Sprinkle with the parsley before serving.

LEEK WITH POTATOES, GARLIC AND THYME

This is soothing and has a helpful effect on the digestive system generally. It's also helpful for COLD RHEUMATISM and for COLDS. Serves 2.

25 *g/1 oz butter or 2 tablespoons olive oil*
1 *onion, peeled and sliced*
1 *garlic clove, peeled and crushed*
½ *teaspoon thyme*
3 *large potatoes, peeled and diced*
2 *leeks, cut into 1 cm/½ in pieces*
sea salt and freshly ground black pepper
chopped fresh parsley

Heat the oil in a deep, heavy-based saucepan. Fry the onion for 5 minutes, then put in the garlic, thyme, potatoes and leeks. Add 200 ml/7 fl oz water and a little salt and stir, then cover and leave to simmer over a gentle heat for 15–20 minutes, or until all the vegetables are tender. Check the seasoning, sprinkle with parsley and serve.

LETTUCE *Lactuca sativa*

Cool, anti-inflammatory, calming, anti-spasmodic

Like cabbage, lettuce can remove inflammation, both internally and externally. Externally, it can be used as a poultice for INFLAMED SWELLINGS

115

and BRUISES; just bind the leaves into position on the affected part and change them every few hours.

Internally, lettuce can be helpful whenever there is inflammation, ulceration or spasms in the digestive system. So ULCERS, GASTRITIS, ULCERATIVE COLITIS and IRRITABLE BOWEL SYNDROME all respond well to this vegetable, especially if it is lightly steamed. Used raw in salads, lettuce is cooling to the system, cleanses the blood and can help CONSTIPATION.

Lettuce has an anti-spasmodic, moistening and loosening action on the lungs, so it may be of value both for DRY COUGHS (where it can create moisture) and for WET COUGHS (where it can loosen the phlegm). For this action it should be combined with an expectorant such as garlic, thyme or ginger.

The ability of lettuce to calm and soothe has been well-known for centuries; lettuce soup is a good remedy for NERVOUS TENSION and INSOMNIA. Lettuce can also reduce sexual desire, especially if combined with marjoram; Pythagoras called it 'the food of the eunuchs'.

Other salad leaves such as endive, chicory and radicchio have similar actions to lettuce, cleansing and cooling the blood, digestive system and the body generally. They do not, however, have such a calming effect on the nervous system and sexual energies. Radicchio, and red varieties of lettuce, can strengthen the blood and tone up the body.

Preparing and Using: Lettuce usually forms the basis of a green salad, but it can also be a starting-point for many variations. For instance, you could add any of the other salad leaves, including some bitter ones (dandelion, in particular, for flavour as well as its extraordinary healing qualities); lightly cooked green beans or mangetouts; bean or alfalfa sprouts; sliced, ripe avocado; nuts or seeds (pine nuts and walnuts, with walnut oil to dress the salad, perhaps) are especially good; tiny cubes of bread (if allowed on your diet), nuts or garlicky chick peas quickly fried in oil and tossed in at the end, all sizzling . . . Such a salad can be served alone or with another salad, such as grated carrot, as a refreshing and healthy accompaniment to a main course. Or, perhaps served with a baked potato, creamy mashed potato or buttered new potatoes, some hot cooked brown rice or millet or OATCAKES (page 160), it can be a substantial, health-giving main course.

Although usually served raw, lettuce is also delicious cooked, and it is more appropriate for some conditions in this form. Cook it lightly, in a steamer, or as described for spinach (page 133); or try the recipes below.

SUMMER LETTUCE SOUP

Serves 4.

> 1 tablespoon olive oil
> 1 onion, peeled and chopped
> 750 g/1½ lb potatoes, peeled and diced
> 450 g/1 lb outside leaves of lettuce
> 1 litre/1¾ pints stock or water
> sea salt and freshly ground black pepper
> single cream (optional)
> chopped fresh herbs (optional)

Heat the oil in a large saucepan, then put in the onion and potatoes. Stir, then cover and cook over a gentle heat for 5 minutes, stirring from time to time. Add the lettuce, cover and cook for a further 5 minutes, then pour in the stock or water, bring to the boil, and simmer for about 15 minutes, until the vegetables are cooked. Liquidise. Season to taste with salt and pepper, reheat, and add a dash of cream and chopped fresh herbs if using.

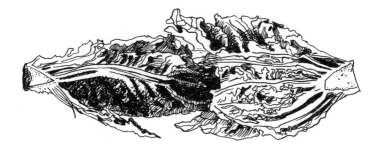

BRAISED LETTUCE HEART WITH MINT

Served with well-cooked brown rice, or with new potatoes, and perhaps a little steamed tofu, this makes a most soothing meal. If a plainer dish is required, leave out the butter, and add an extra 2 tablespoons water to the pan. Serves 2–4.

> 25 g/1 oz butter
> 1 hearty lettuce, cut into thick wedges
> sea salt
> 1–2 tablespoons chopped fresh mint

Melt the butter, without browning, in a large saucepan, then add the lettuce wedges, 2 tablespoons water and a little salt. Sauté gently for 1–2 minutes, turning the lettuce wedges until they are coated with the butter. Cover the pan, and let the lettuce continue to cook for about 5 minutes, or until tender. Add the mint, check the seasoning, and serve.

NETTLES *Urtica dioica*

Warm, tonic, astringent

Nettles make a fine, warming tonic, raising the yang energy and providing an abundance of vitamins and minerals, including iron, silica, potassium and vitamins A and C. They are especially helpful for people who are weak and pale and suffer from ANAEMIA; they cleanse and purify the blood and can help BRITTLE BONES because of their silica content. They are also useful for COLD RHEUMATISM, the type of condition which has cramping pains and is worse in cold weather. Nettles strengthen lax tissues in the intestines and stop DIARRHOEA; they are also helpful in stemming EXCESS URINATION, and, for this condition, can be taken both by the elderly and by children. An infusion of nettles is good as a hair rinse (see page 236).

Preparing and Using: Wearing gloves, pick tender stinging nettles from an unpolluted spot. They can be used to make a tea or decoction; they can be cooked like spinach (page 133); or they can be made into a delicious soup, see below.

VELVETY NETTLE SOUP

Delicately flavoured and velvety green, this soup is much better than the humble ingredients would lead you to imagine. It's good to eat as it is, and even better with a dollop of cream swirled into each portion. Serves 4.

> 1 *tablespoon olive oil*
> 1 *onion, peeled and chopped*
> 450 *g/1 lb potatoes, peeled and diced*
> 225 *g/8 oz tender nettles*
> *sea salt and freshly ground black pepper*
> *freshly grated nutmeg*
> *single cream (optional)*

Heat the oil in a large saucepan, then put in the onion and potatoes. Stir, then cover and cook over a gentle heat for 5 minutes, stirring from time to time. Add the nettles, cover and cook for a further 5 minutes, then pour in 1 litre/1¾ pints water, bring to the boil, and simmer for about 15 minutes, until the vegetables are cooked. Liquidise. Season to taste with salt, pepper and nutmeg, reheat, and add the cream if using.

ONION *Allium coepa*

Hot, expectorant, tonic, diuretic

Like garlic, onions have warming, expectorant, antiseptic and tonic properties. Research has shown that onions can have an anti-bacterial action, helping RESPIRATORY, DIGESTIVE and URINARY INFECTIONS. For the latter, the diuretic quality of onions is also helpful, cleansing the kidneys and bladder; and, for the same reason, onions are useful for WEIGHT LOSS.

Onions are valuable for many other conditions: for COLDS AND FLU when there is shivering and blocked nose and sinuses; also for BRONCHITIS and ASTHMA with mucus. They're recommended for DIABETES and HYPOGLYCAEMIA; for COLD RHEUMATISM with swollen joints and cramping pains which are worse in cold, damp weather; and also as a general stimulant and tonic, raising the yang energy (useful for those who are cold and debilitated).

Research has shown that onions can help cleanse the blood and reduce the level of cholesterol, thus reducing the risk of HEART DISEASE and BLOOD CLOTS. In addition, onions have a cleansing effect on the lymphatic system, helping to clear congested lymph glands and thus heal SKIN PROBLEMS.

Cooked onions, like leeks, are useful for CONSTIPATION and inflammation in the digestive tract. When cooked, they lose much of their heat and antibiotic properties but become more soothing for COUGHS, DIGESTIVE INFLAMMATIONS and spasms.

Note: Like any hot substance, onions should not be used when there is excessive heat in the system, especially if this is in the digestive system and associated with GASTRITIS and ULCERS.

Preparing and Using: Onions vary a good deal in their pungency; large, Spanish onions are often particularly mild, and delicious both raw and cooked. They can be baked or steamed; boiled, fried or made into wonderfully soothing soups. To bake them, trim but don't skin large

119

onions. Put them on a baking sheet and bake at 200°C/400°F/Gas Mark 6 for about 1 hour, until they feel soft. When they're done, split them and serve with butter, salt and pepper.

BROWN ONION SOUP

A warming, comforting soup for COLDS and chills of the shivery kind. Serves 4.

> *2 tablespoons olive oil*
> *1 kg/2 lb onions, peeled and thinly sliced*
> *900 ml/1½ pints stock or water*
> *2 garlic cloves, peeled and crushed*
> *lemon juice*
> *sea salt and freshly ground black pepper*
> *chopped parsley or chives*

Heat the oil in a large saucepan, then fry the onions for 30 minutes until they're soft and a deep golden brown, but don't let them burn. Add the stock or water, garlic, and a few drops of lemon juice. Bring the soup to the boil and let it simmer for about 10 minutes. Season to taste with salt and pepper, sprinkle over the chopped parsley or chives, and serve.

CREAMY ONION SOUP

Serves 4.

> *2 tablespoons olive oil or butter*
> *750 g/1½ lb onions, peeled and thinly sliced*
> *1 large potato, peeled and diced*
> *salt and freshly ground black pepper*
> *freshly grated nutmeg*
> *single cream (optional)*

Heat half the oil or butter in a large saucepan, then put in a third of the onion and all the potato. Stir, then cover and cook without browning over a gentle heat for 10 minutes, stirring from time to time. Add 1 litre/1¾ pints water, bring to the boil, then simmer for about 15 minutes, until the vegetables are cooked. Meanwhile, heat the remaining oil or butter in another pan and fry the rest of the onion very gently, with a lid on the pan, for about 15 minutes, until tender, but, again, not browned. Liquidise the potato soup mixture, then add the fried onion.

Season to taste with salt, pepper and nutmeg, reheat, and add the cream if using.

PEA *Pisum sativum*

Neutral, nutrient, laxative

Like potatoes and grains, peas provide a good source of energy. They strengthen the stomach and its lining, helping an OVERHEATED DIGESTION. Like leeks and artichokes, they have a good laxative action, so they are useful for CONSTIPATION; they also have a mild diuretic action, helping to eliminate OEDEMA (FLUID RETENTION). Some authors recommend peas as a mild aid for DIABETES and HYPOGLYCAEMIA.

Dried peas have similar qualities in a more concentrated form, and provide useful amounts of B vitamins. They can make an excellent soup, or a purée for serving with other vegetables (see recipes under **Pulses**, page 147).

Preparing and Using: Fresh peas, bought in the pod, are a delight if you can get them when they are young and fresh enough for the peas to be tender. Otherwise frozen peas are the best bet, and are particularly good cooked with lettuce, or as a smooth soup (see recipes below). Alternatively, you could use sugarsnap peas or mangetout, which can be cooked whole in a little boiling water, steamed or added to stir-fries at the last minute: they only take a few seconds to cook.

PEAS COOKED WITH LETTUCE

If you are using fresh peas for this, you will need about 1.5 kg/3 lb before podding. Serves 4.

> *25 g/1 oz butter*
> *8 outside lettuce leaves*
> *450 g/1 lb shelled fresh peas or frozen peas*
> *3 sprigs of fresh mint*
> *sea salt*

Melt half the butter in a saucepan, then put in the lettuce leaves. Put the peas on top of the lettuce, then add the rest of the butter, 2 tablespoons water and the mint. Cover and leave to cook over a gentle heat for 5–10 minutes, or until the peas are tender. Season to taste with a little sea salt.

121

GREEN PEA SOUP WITH MINT

Serves 4.

> 25 g/1 oz butter
> 1 onion, peeled and chopped
> 225 g/8 oz potato, peeled and diced
> 450 g/1 lb frozen peas
> 10 sprigs of fresh mint
> sea salt and freshly ground black pepper
> Barbados sugar
> 150 ml/5 fl oz single cream (optional)

Melt the butter in a large saucepan, and fry the onion gently for 5 minutes. Add the potato, stir well, then cover and cook for a further 5–10 minutes without browning. Add the peas, 600 ml/1 pint water and 5 of the mint sprigs. Bring up to the boil, then cover and cook gently for about 15 minutes, until the potato is tender. Liquidise the soup (including the mint sprigs). Then, for a smooth, velvety texture, pass the soup through a sieve. Season to taste with salt, pepper and a little sugar. Serve hot or cold, with a swirl of cream on top if you like, and the rest of the mint snipped over the top.

POTATO *Solanum tuberosum*

Neutral, nourishing, anti-inflammatory

Potatoes are both nourishing and anti-inflammatory. Their juice, in particular, has a healing effect on ULCERS and inflammations of the digestive tract, such as ULCERATIVE COLITIS and DIVERTICULITIS. For this purpose, the juice can be mixed with cabbage juice (see page 96). Whether the juice is mixed or taken on its own, the treatment is half a cup, twice a day, after main meals.

Mixed in equal parts with courgettes, potatoes have a soothing effect on the urinary system, helping to eliminate EXCESS URINATION and relieve KIDNEY INFLAMMATION. On their own or mixed with other anti-inflammatory vegetables, in soups or other dishes, potatoes also have a calming effect on the respiratory system, relieving irritation and COUGHS.

Potatoes are popularly believed to be fattening. However, although they can help to build the body up when required, if they are baked or boiled and eaten with salad or cooked vegetables, they can be a good source of energy and vitamins without causing obesity. It's when they're fried in large amounts of fat – particularly saturated fat – that they can add on the inches, but this has much more to do with the fat than the potatoes.

Valnet, the renowned French naturopathic doctor and researcher, recommends potatoes for sugar disorders such as DIABETES and HYPO-GLYCAEMIA.

The juice of raw grated potatoes can be applied externally, and is helpful for INFLAMMATIONS, SWELLINGS and CYSTS, as are cabbage, lettuce, marshmallow and marigold.

Note: Excessive consumption of stodgy foods such as potatoes can cause sluggishness in some people.

Preparing and Using: Scrape or peel potatoes, or scrub the skins and leave them on. Boil in enough water to cover until tender and serve with butter, or mash with butter and milk or cream until light and fluffy, or choose large potatoes, prick and bake at 230°C/450°F/Gas Mark 8, for 1–1½ hours until they feel soft. Sweet potatoes are delicious for a change and can be prepared in a similar way; just scrub, cut into pieces, and bake like potatoes; or peel, boil and purée.

One of the easiest and best ways of cooking this vegetable, BIRCHER POTATOES, is named after the renowned German naturopath and inventor of muesli, Bircher-Benner. Scrub the potatoes, cut them in half, then put them cut-side down on an oiled baking sheet. Sprinkle with caraway, aniseed or cumin seeds, and bake at 200°C/400°F/Gas Mark 6 for 45–60 minutes, until the potatoes are soft and the cut sides are golden brown and crisp.

LAYERED POTATO BAKE

This makes a healthy and delicious main course when served with a large green salad or a cooked leafy green vegetable such as spinach. Serves 2–3.

> *3 tablespoons olive oil or 40 g/1½ oz butter*
> *1 kg/2 lb potatoes, peeled and cut into thin slices (no thicker than 5 mm/¼ in)*
> *1 onion, peeled and very thinly sliced*
> *1–2 garlic cloves, peeled and crushed*
> *sea salt*
> *freshly grated nutmeg*

Preheat the oven to 220°C/425°F/Gas Mark 7. Brush a shallow oven-proof dish with 1 tablespoon oil or 15 g/½ oz butter. Put the potatoes and onion into a saucepan containing 2.5 cm/1 in water; bring to the boil and simmer for 8 minutes, or until the potatoes are just tender, and most of the water has been absorbed. Add the garlic and season to taste with salt and nutmeg. Spoon the mixture into the prepared dish and level the top. Pour the rest of the oil, or put small pieces of the remaining butter, over the top. Bake for about 30 minutes, or until browned and crisp on top.

See also LEEK WITH POTATOES, GARLIC AND THYME (page 115), CABBAGE AND POTATO SOUP WITH THYME AND FENNEL (page 97) and BUBBLE AND SQUEAK (page 98).

PUMPKIN *Cucurbita*

Neutral to cooling, anti-inflammatory

Pumpkin has a soothing and cooling action on the stomach; in the terminology of Chinese medicine, it 'nourishes the yin of the stomach'. It is helpful not only with the usual symptoms of INDIGESTION such as bloating and flatulence, but also with burning, acidity and hot flushes which are worse after eating hot and spicy food. A soup of pumpkin, courgettes, carrots and sage (see below) soothes and heals such hot symptoms, including hot flushes and night sweats. This soup should be taken daily for a while, until the symptoms ease and strength returns.

Chronic GASTRIC FLU, with feverishness and an upset stomach, responds well to a pumpkin, courgette and carrot soup, but in this case you should add ½ teaspoon cinnamon and a small piece of vanilla pod. This same soup, but with a pinch of fennel and aniseed and, if possible, some fresh mint leaves, can be used to take away excessive heat in the digestive system which leads to conditions such as ULCERS, GASTRITIS and ULCERATIVE COLITIS.

Pumpkin has been found valuable for spasms, irritation and inflammation of the respiratory tract, and illnesses such as ASTHMA. For these, the pumpkin, courgette and carrot soup is also excellent, but this time with the addition of some sage and marjoram.

Preparing and Using: Peel the pumpkin, remove the seeds and cut the flesh into even-sized pieces. Pumpkin can be steamed or boiled, braised, stir-fried or made into a soup.

One of the simplest and best ways of cooking pumpkin is to braise it in butter. Just put the prepared pumpkin into a heavy-based saucepan with 15 g/½ oz butter, 4 tablespoons water and a little sea salt. Cover and cook gently until tender – about 10–15 minutes.

PUMPKIN AND TOFU PURÉE

This is a smooth, creamy purée, nourishing and good to eat as a main course when little else appeals, perhaps accompanied by some well-cooked plain brown rice. If garlic is recommended for your condition, this can be puréed, raw, with the pumpkin, or cooked with the pumpkin then puréed. Other spices can be added as desired, particularly those which are helpful to the digestion such as cardamom, cloves, aniseed, coriander and caraway. Pumpkin and cardamom purée is particularly delicious, and if sweetened with a dash of apple juice concentrate, it can be eaten as a pudding. Serve the savoury version with carrots and courgettes as vegetables – the contrasting colours are attractive – plus cooked brown rice, maize or millet, for a mixture which is helpful for an OVERHEATED DIGESTION. Serves 3–4.

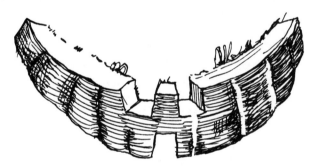

450 g/1 lb pumpkin (weighed after removing skin and seeds),
    diced
275 g/10 oz firm tofu, drained
2 garlic cloves, peeled (optional)
sea salt
freshly ground black pepper (optional)
freshly grated nutmeg (optional)

Boil or steam the pumpkin until tender, and drain if necessary, reserving the liquid. Purée the pumpkin and tofu in a food processor until smooth and creamy (the mixture will look curdled at first, but will become smooth as you continue). Add 1–2 tablespoons reserved cooking liquid if necessary, to get a soft consistency. Add the garlic cloves, if using, and whizz again. Season to taste with salt, and pepper and nutmeg if using.

PUMPKIN, COURGETTE AND CARROT SOUP

A wonderfully soothing soup; good for COLITIS and ULCERS. Serves 4.

> *25 g/1 oz butter or 2 tablespoons olive oil*
> *225 g/8 oz pumpkin (weighed after removing skin and seeds),*
>   *diced*
> *225 g/8 oz carrots, scraped and diced*
> *225 g/8 oz courgettes, sliced*
> *½–1 teaspoon dried sage or 2–3 teaspoons chopped fresh sage*
> *sea salt*

Heat the butter or oil in a large saucepan, and add the pumpkin and carrots. Stir, then cover and cook gently for 10 minutes, stirring from time to time. Add 1 litre/1¾ pints water, bring to the boil, then simmer gently for a further 15 minutes or so, until the vegetables are almost tender. Add the courgettes and sage, and cook for a further 3–5 minutes, until all the vegetables are cooked. Season lightly with salt. This soup can be served as it is with chunky pieces of vegetable; or it can be partially liquidised, so that there are some chunks of vegetable in a creamy base; or wholly liquidised to a creamy consistency.

See also CABBAGE, PUMPKIN, FENNEL AND CARROT SOUP WITH ANISEED (page 97).

RADISHES *Raphanus spp*

Neutral with warming potential, stimulant, expectorant

There are several types of radish, all of which have useful healing properties. Like mint, they are both warming and cooling; they seem hot when you eat them, but leave a feeling of coolness. This is especially true after they have been boiled or steamed. The pungent quality of raw radishes acts primarily on the respiratory system, helping to get rid of phlegm, to clear BLOCKED SINUSES and to expel COLDS generally. Radishes drain and cleanse an OVERHEATED LIVER and DIGESTION and help to clear CONSTIPATION. Being diuretic, they also help the body to get rid of excess fluid.

The black radish is a long, black-skinned radish, well-known in France and southern Europe where it is valued for its ability to cleanse and regenerate the liver. It is widely prescribed by French naturopaths for this purpose. Mooli is a long, white radish which is much used in India. It has the same liver-strengthening properties as the black radish, and is also very good for constipation. The familiar pink or red radish shares all the main properties described for the others but in a milder form. For horseradish, which belongs to a different family, but which has similar properties, see under **Flowers, Herbs and Spices**, page 63.

Note: Radishes should not be taken when there is an excess of heat or inflammation in the body, especially in the digestive system, as in GASTRITIS or ULCERS.

Preparing and Using: The radishes should look fresh and crisp. Scrub, then slice, dice or coarsely grate the larger radishes; the little red ones can of course be left whole. All radishes can be eaten raw or cooked; if you are cooking them, they are best lightly steamed or added to stir-fries at the last minute so that they retain their crispness.

The red radishes, in particular, make a pretty addition to salads and are particularly good with dips, especially if they have their leaves still attached (these can be eaten, too). Try a salad of sliced radishes mixed with oranges and watercress; slices of radish and cucumber; radishes and lightly cooked sweetcorn; stir-fried mooli and carrot, both cut into thin matchsticks; or grated mooli and apple, mixed together and served with lettuce or watercress.

SEAWEEDS

Cold, cleansing, diuretic

Edible types of seaweed with therapeutic properties include kombu, kelp, nori, wakame, arame, hiziki and bladderwrack. Seaweeds have many beneficial actions, perhaps the most important being their ability to cleanse the blood of toxins, including, research suggests, heavy metals such as strontium and barium. It is thought that this is because they contain olginic acid which binds these metals and enables them to be eliminated from the body. Some authors claim that, like miso, seaweeds can even help remove the effects of radiation.

Their cleansing properties make seaweeds particularly valuable for

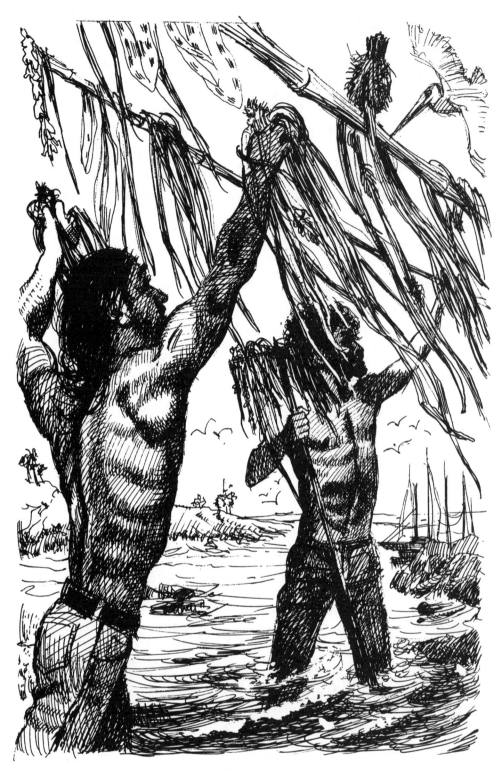

Drying seaweed

SKIN INFLAMMATIONS where the painful areas are red, swollen and pussy. They are also effective in cleansing the lymphatic system and dispersing swollen lymph nodules. Seaweeds increase urination and help to eliminate fats and mucus from the body; they are very helpful in cases of OEDEMA (FLUID RETENTION).

Seaweeds make the blood more alkaline, thus helping to counteract the acid-forming effects of eating meat, sugar and refined carbohydrates. They are extremely rich in minerals and vitamins, and therefore useful when extra nutrients are needed. Their rich iodine content makes seaweeds particularly valuable when there is mild HYPOTHYROIDISM and GENERAL LETHARGY.

Note: Seaweed should not be used more than once a week in cases of HYPERTHYROIDISM with its associated symptoms of palpitations, restlessness, weight loss, poor sleep, and so on. Also, prolonged use of seaweeds is not advisable for people who lack yang energy, giving a feeling of low energy, and causing weight loss, coldness, weakness and pallor.

Preparing and Using: Some types of seaweed, such as kelp and bladderwrack, are best taken in tablet form. Healthfood shops and wholefood stores do, however, stock several seaweeds which can be delicious. Only a very small quantity of dried seaweed is needed because it expands considerably once rehydrated. Simply wash the seaweed to remove excess salt and any sand, then soak it in water for a few minutes. Some types of seaweed – wakame, for instance – have tough stems, so these should be cut out. Then the seaweed can be shredded, if necessary, and either used raw, or simmered in water for up to 30 minutes, until really tender.

Seaweed can be added to salads and stir-fries or made into soups. A piece of kombu seaweed added to pulses at the beginning of cooking is supposed to help make them tender. Vegetarian jelling agents (to replace gelatine) are made from seaweed, and are available in flake or powdered forms. They are valuable for their anti-inflammatory and cooling properties. See the recipe for PINEAPPLE JELLY (page 197).

For a delicious salad, soak some pieces of wakame in water until soft. Cut out the tough stems, shred the wakame and sprinkle with wine vinegar, rice vinegar or lemon juice to taste (rice vinegar is best if vinegar is allowed in your diet), a dash of a good soy sauce such as shoyu, a little honey and a pinch of sea salt if needed. Some hot spices such as chilli are good (unless you have an inflamed condition) – I sometimes add

129

1–2 dried red chillies, for quite a fiery salad – and some sliced onion and garlic. Leave to marinate for as long as is convenient. This is good as a nibble on its own or with plain brown rice with or without some STIR-FRIED VEGETABLES WITH FRESH GINGER (page 99), some LIME-MARINATED TOFU WITH CHILLI AND BLACK PEPPER (page 150) and a sprinkling of sesame salt or GOMASIO (page 172).

CLEANSING SEAWEED SOUP

Serves 4.

> 3–4 *pieces wakame*
> 1 *tablespoon olive oil*
> 1 *onion, peeled and chopped*
> 225 *g/8 oz carrots, scrubbed and sliced*
> 4 *celery sticks, chopped*
> 1–2 *teaspoons miso*

Wash the wakame, then cover it with water and leave to soften for a few minutes. When it is flexible, cut out the tough stems and chop the wakame. Heat the oil in a large saucepan and sauté the onion for 5 minutes, then add the carrots and celery, and cook for a further 5 minutes. Add the wakame and 1 litre/1¾ pints water, bring to the boil, cover and simmer for 10–15 minutes, until the vegetables are tender. Stir in the miso, to taste, and serve immediately.

WAKAME OMELETTE

> 2 *pieces wakame*
> 1 *egg, beaten*
> 2 *teaspoons olive oil*
> *soy sauce*
> *sesame seeds*

Wash the wakame, then cover it with water and leave to soften for a few minutes. When it is flexible, cut out the tough stems, shred the wakame and mix it with the egg. Heat the oil in a frying pan, then pour in the wakame mixture, stirring gently until set. Roll the omelette up and cut into pieces. Serve hot or cold, dipping the pieces first in soy sauce and then in sesame seeds before eating.

VEGETABLE SALAD WITH WAKAME

This salad has a Chinese feel to it and is good with some well-cooked brown rice. Serves 1–2.

2 pieces wakame
2 carrots, scraped and sliced diagonally
a 2.5–5 cm/1–2 in piece of mooli, sliced diagonally
100 g/4 oz cabbage, shredded
a 2.5–5 cm/1–2 in piece of cucumber, peeled and sliced
1 teaspoon honey
1 tablespoon rice vinegar, wine vinegar or lemon juice
1 tablespoon shoyu
sea salt

Wash the wakame, then cover it with water and leave to soften for a few minutes. When it is flexible, cut out the tough stems, shred the wakame, and put it in a bowl. Steam the carrots and mooli until they begin to get tender, then add the cabbage and steam until all the vegetables are just tender but still with plenty of bite. Add them to the wakame, along with the cucumber, honey, vinegar or lemon juice and shoyu. Mix well and season with sea salt if needed. Leave to marinate for about 30 minutes, stirring from time to time.

HIZIKI SALAD

Hiziki, or arame, which look a bit alike, just need rinsing and soaking for a few minutes before being added to vegetable salads, although you can cook them for a few minutes in boiling water if you want to make them more tender. Some hot brown rice goes well with this salad, turning it into a complete light meal. You could also serve some GINGER-MARINATED TOFU (page 149) and some sesame salt or GOMASIO (page 172). Serves 1–2.

a few pieces of hiziki or arame
a 2.5–5 cm/1–2 in piece mooli or a small bunch of radishes
corn from 1 sweetcorn cob or 75 g/3 oz frozen sweetcorn kernels
a 2.5–5 cm/1–2 in piece of cucumber, peeled and sliced
1 teaspoon honey
1 tablespoon rice vinegar, wine vinegar or lemon juice
1 tablespoon shoyu
sea salt

Soak the hiziki or arame in water while you prepare the rest of the ingredients. Slice the mooli, or trim and slice the radishes, and put into a bowl. The corn can be used raw or lightly steamed for 2–3 minutes. Add this to the radishes, along with the cucumber, honey, vinegar or lemon juice and shoyu. Drain the hiziki or arame and add that too, mixing well. Season with a little sea salt if needed, then leave to marinate for about 30 minutes, stirring from time to time.

SHIITAKE MUSHROOMS *Lentinus edodes*

Neutral

The shiitake mushroom is an Eastern fungus which grows on the wood of dead deciduous trees. A great deal of research in China and Japan suggests that this mushroom, and the raishi mushroom, are valuable in strengthening the immune system, and helping to prevent the growth of tumours in CANCER. Shiitake mushrooms can be bought dried in Oriental shops and some healthfood shops; or, increasingly, they are available fresh in supermarkets.

Preparing and Using: Soak dried mushrooms in water for 30 minutes, then drain and add to stir-fries, soups and vegetable casseroles. Fresh shiitake mushrooms are prepared in the same way as ordinary fresh mushrooms; just wash them and slice if necessary. They can be lightly sautéed in butter or oil, perhaps with some garlic added; and they are an excellent addition to any stir-fry or vegetable mixture. Try them on toast; as a filling for an omelette; or in any of your favourite mushroom dishes. They have a firmer texture than ordinary mushrooms and a delicious, distinctive flavour.

SHIITAKE MUSHROOMS IN SOY SAUCE WITH SESAME SEEDS

This is delicious as a first course with some warm rolls or toast; or you could serve it with boiled rice and some stir-fried cabbage or mixed vegetables. Serves 4.

> *450 g/1 lb shiitake mushrooms, or a mixture of shiitake and ordinary mushrooms*
> *2 tablespoons olive oil*

2 teaspoons cornflour
4 tablespoons tamari or shoyu
sea salt and freshly ground black pepper
1 tablespoon sesame seeds

Wash, dry and slice the mushrooms. Heat the oil in a saucepan and add the mushrooms; fry for about 5 minutes, or until tender and heated through (shiitake mushrooms never get very soft). Mix the cornflour with the tamari or shoyu and add to the pan; stir until the liquid has thickened. Season to taste (you may not need any salt at all because of the soy sauce) and serve sprinkled with sesame seeds.

SPINACH *Spinacia oleracea*

Cooling, tonic

Spinach is considered to have a strengthening and vitalising effect on the whole body. Its high iron and mineral content makes it a very good blood-builder; it also cools and clears the blood, and is therefore helpful for SKIN PROBLEMS. Spinach is a mild laxative, useful for CONSTIPATION, and also has diuretic properties. Some Chinese tests suggest that, like carrots, fennel and bilberries, spinach can strengthen the eyesight.

Note: Because of its high oxalic acid content, spinach (like tomatoes, peanuts, tea, rhubarb, oranges, chocolate and strawberries) is not advised if you suffer from KIDNEY STONES or RHEUMATISM.

Preparing and Using: Wash spinach 3 times in bowlfuls of cold water, then cook it in a large saucepan without added water. Use the end of a fish slice to push it down and chop it while it cooks. It takes 7–10 minutes. Drain and add butter, salt, freshly ground black pepper and freshly grated nutmeg. For a more substantial dish, you could add some curd cheese and grated cheese to cooked spinach, put it in a shallow heatproof dish, sprinkle with more grated cheese and brown under the grill.

Spinach is excellent as a filling for pancakes or lasagne, and can be made into light soufflés and roulades. It blends well with lentils, particularly the brown type, and can be made into a good soup (see below).

Tender leaves of spinach make a pleasant, sharp-tasting addition to a salad bowl.

SPINACH SOUP

Serves 4.

> 1 *tablespoon olive oil*
> 1 *onion, peeled and chopped*
> 750 *g/1½ lb potatoes, peeled and diced*
> 450 *g/1 lb spinach*
> 900 *ml/1½ pints stock or water*
> *sea salt and freshly ground black pepper*
> *freshly grated nutmeg*
> *single cream (optional)*

Heat the oil in a large saucepan, and put in the onion and potatoes. Stir, then cover and cook over a gentle heat for 5 minutes, stirring from time to time. Add the spinach, cover and cook for a further 5 minutes, then pour in the stock or water, bring to the boil, and simmer for about 15 minutes, until the vegetables are cooked. Liquidise. Season with salt, pepper and freshly grated nutmeg. Reheat, and add the cream if using.

SPINACH WITH CUMIN SEEDS

Serve this with some brown rice, SPICY LENTIL DAL (page 144) and perhaps some CUCUMBER RAITA WITH FRESH MINT (page 107) for a complete meal. Serves 2–4.

> 1 *kg/2 lb fresh spinach, thoroughly washed*
> 2 *onions, peeled and sliced*
> 2 *tablespoons olive oil*
> 1 *garlic clove, peeled and crushed*
> 2 *teaspoons cumin seeds*
> *sea salt*

Put the spinach, which should be still damp, into a large saucepan without any extra water. Cover and cook for 8–10 minutes, or until the spinach is tender, then drain thoroughly. Meanwhile, fry the onions in the oil for 7–8 minutes, until almost tender, then add the garlic and cumin and cook for a further 2–3 minutes. Add the spinach, mix, season with salt to taste, and serve.

TOMATO *Lycopersicum esculentum*

Cooling, cleansing

Tomatoes cool and strengthen, as well as supplying many vitamins and minerals. They aid digestion and, like cucumber, facilitate the assimilation of fatty and spicy dishes such as curries, oily pasta and fried foods. They are both a laxative, thus useful for CONSTIPATION, and a diuretic, eliminating excess fluid from the system.

Like lettuce, watercress, endive and cucumber, tomatoes cool and cleanse the blood, easing SKIN INFLAMMATIONS. They also help to lower cholesterol and are believed to help conditions such as HYPERTENSION (HIGH BLOOD PRESSURE), often indicated by a red face and bloodshot eyes.

Other salads, hot vegetables and spices such as garlic and onions, and fresh herbs such as mint and basil, all combine well with tomatoes.

Note: Because of their oxalic acid content, tomatoes are not advised if you suffer from KIDNEY STONES or acute RHEUMATISM.

Preparing and Using: Firm tomatoes can be sliced as they are, without skinning, unless you particularly wish to eat them with the skins removed. For a simple but very tasty tomato salad, slice about 450 g/1 lb tomatoes, put them in a dish and sprinkle with sea salt and freshly ground black pepper. Pour over the juice of half a lemon and 1–2 tablespoons good olive oil. If possible, leave for 30 minutes or so for the flavours to blend. Some torn fresh basil leaves are a classic addition to this salad, and delicious, as is some thinly sliced raw onion. See also FENNEL AND TOMATO VINAIGRETTE WITH BLACK OLIVES (page 111).

WATERCRESS *Nasturtium officinale*

Neutral to slightly warming, tonic, cleansing

Watercress, especially raw, is highly recommended for people who are debilitated, with EMPTY OR WEAK BLOOD (ANAEMIA), giving symptoms such as paleness, dizziness, weak nails and brittle hair. This is because watercress is rich in minerals like iron, potassium, calcium, sulphur and phosphorus, and in vitamins, particularly the B group (including folic acid), carotene and vitamin C. Together with dandelions and nettles, watercress is one of the most nutritious vegetables.

Recommended for strengthening the pancreas and therefore helpful in DIABETES and HYPOGLYCAEMIA, watercress also cleanses the lymphatic system, especially in weak, anaemic people. It strengthens the natural defences and the lungs, helps to get rid of excess fluid and eases RHEUMATISM. According to Dr Binet, watercress may also have some effect against CANCER.

Pulverised to a paste and applied to the hair for 2 hours before being washed off; or made into a tea and used as a wash after shampooing, watercress (like rosemary and nettles) strengthens the scalp, stimulates hair growth and may help to counteract HAIR LOSS.

Note: In some cases watercress can aggravate CYSTITIS.

Preparing and Using: Watercress should always be bought from a reliable source (not picked from a stream or river because of the danger of liver fluke), and washed thoroughly before eating. It is usually eaten raw or as a soup, but can be cooked quickly in a dry pan until wilted. Watercress is also excellent in sandwiches made from thin wholemeal bread – a good lunch or supper dish with or without a light soup.

WATERCRESS SOUP

A cleansing, diuretic soup, good for RHEUMATISM and OEDEMA (FLUID RETENTION). Serves 4.

> 1 tablespoon olive oil
> 1 onion, peeled and chopped
> 750 g/1½ lb potatoes, peeled and diced
> 1 litre/1¾ pints stock or water
> a bunch of watercress
> sea salt and freshly ground black pepper
> single cream (optional)

Heat the oil in a large saucepan, and put in the onion and potato. Stir, then cover and cook over a gentle heat for 10 minutes, stirring from time to time. Add the stock or water, cover, bring to the boil, then simmer for about 15 minutes, until the vegetables are cooked. Liquidise with the watercress. Return to the saucepan. Season with salt and pepper, then reheat gently. This is good with some single cream stirred into it, if you wish.

Pulses

Pulses are an excellent source of protein and energy, especially for vegetarians or semi-vegetarians. They combine well with grains; their amino acid patterns complement each other so that when eaten together each provides more protein than it can on its own.

Rich in fibre, pulses have a laxative action which makes them useful in treating CONSTIPATION. They are also reputed to be slightly diuretic. They are mainly neutral to cooling, with tofu (made from soya beans) probably being the coolest and lentils the warmest.

Some people find pulses indigestible and flatulence-causing, particularly when they first start eating them, perhaps after many years of eating meat. If this is a problem, make sure that you cook them carefully as described below. Adding wind-expelling spices can greatly reduce the problem. The best ones are fennel, bay, oregano, ginger, thyme, cloves, mint, cumin, caraway, coriander, tarragon and savory – there are plenty to choose from! Start by eating small quantities of pulses to find how much you can eat at a time without problems, then gradually increase the amount. An average-size serving of pulses would be about 25–50 g/1–2 oz (dry weight).

BUYING AND STORING

Although a number of pulses can be bought in cans, ready to use, we prefer the dried ones which you soak and cook yourself. They are certainly a great deal cheaper. Buy them in small amounts and keep them in a cool, dry place. The longer they are stored, the harder pulses get, and the cooking time will vary accordingly.

COOKING

Put the beans or lentils in a bowl, cover them with cold water and leave to soak for several hours. Or put them in a large saucepan, cover with water, bring to the boil, then remove from the heat, cover and leave to soak for 1 hour. Drain and rinse the pulses, then put them in a pan with 3 times their volume in cold water and bring to the boil. Boil rapidly, without a lid on the pan, for 10 minutes. Then cover, reduce the heat, and simmer gently until tender, topping up the water from time to time if necessary.

Most beans cook in 1¼–1½ hours. The exceptions are red lentils, which take 20 minutes; mung beans and split peas, which take about 40 minutes; and chick peas which can take anything from an unusually quick 40 minutes to a more typical 2–3 hours. If you want to use a pressure cooker to cut the cooking time, you can omit the 10 minutes of rapid boiling and simply cook the beans at high pressure for a third of their normal cooking time.

Some recipes incorporate the beans after they have been soaked and they cook slowly with the other ingredients. Beans absorb flavours well this way but be careful not to add salt or acid ingredients (such as tomatoes or vinegar) which can prevent them from softening properly.

Cooked beans freeze well. The mushy type, like lentils, need to be frozen in containers in suitably sized portions. The type which keep their shape, like red kidney beans, can be spread out on a tray to freeze, then put into a polythene bag or large container so that you can take out the amount you need, as you do with frozen peas or sweetcorn.

Cooked beans can be made into a variety of dishes: sautéed gently in a little oil with onions, vegetables and spices to make simple and delicious vegetable mixtures; mashed, combined with fried onion and garlic, formed into burgers and fried or baked; or mixed with chopped fresh herbs, olive oil and fresh lemon juice or wine vinegar to make a fragrant salad.

SPROUTING

Sprouting pulses increases their nutritional value and, some people find, makes them more digestible. Simply rinse a couple of heaped tablespoons of your chosen variety – mung beans, whole lentils, aduki beans, chick peas, and alfalfa seeds are some of the most successful – in an old sieve or colander. Rinse them twice a day until the beans or seeds have sprouted. This takes 2–5 days, depending on the type and the temperature. Once they have sprouted, you can arrest further development by storing them in the fridge, where they will keep for 2–3 days. They are a delicious and health-giving addition to sandwiches, salads or stir-fries. Any beans which haven't sprouted are surprisingly hard, so watch your teeth when eating them.

ADUKI BEAN *Phaseolus angularis*

Neutral

Aduki beans strengthen the pancreas and are therefore useful in DIABETES and HYPOGLYCAEMIA. They remove excess water from the system

138

and strengthen the kidneys, and also help to reduce lymphatic swellings, especially when combined with seaweeds and onions.

Preparing and Using: Aduki beans take about 40–50 minutes to cook after soaking. They are often prepared with a piece of seaweed, as in the recipe below, which reduces the time they take to cook, improves their flavour and is said to make them more digestible. They are particularly good in soups and are improved with the addition of sweet ingredients and spices: carrots, ginger, cinnamon, a dash of sugar, honey or apple juice concentrate.

ADUKI BEANS WITH ONIONS, CARROTS AND GINGER

Serves 4.

> 225 g/8 oz aduki beans
> 1 piece kombu seaweed (optional)
> 2 tablespoons olive oil
> 1 large onion, peeled and chopped
> 2 carrots, scrubbed and coarsely grated
> 1 tablespoon grated fresh ginger
> 2 garlic cloves, peeled and crushed
> sea salt and freshly ground black pepper
> Barbados sugar or honey (optional)

Soak the aduki beans in cold water for about 1 hour. If using kombu, break this into pieces and soak it with the beans. Cook the beans and kombu for 40–50 minutes, until the beans are tender. Heat the oil in a large saucepan and fry the onion for 5 minutes. Then add the carrots, ginger and garlic, and fry for a further 5–10 minutes. Drain the aduki beans of excess water, and add them to the onion mixture. Season to taste with salt, pepper and a dash of sugar or honey if needed.

BROAD BEAN *Vicia faba*

Neutral to cooling

These small round brown beans, sometimes known as 'foul' or 'tic' beans, are available at any Middle Eastern shop. They have an excellent laxative action, almost as good as that of red kidney beans, to ease CONSTIPATION. In addition, some researchers believe they have a tonic

139

effect on the nervous system, which is helpful for conditions ranging from simple TENSION and NERVOUS STRESS to more complex problems such as MYALGIC ENCEPHALOMYELITIS (ME) and MULTIPLE SCLEROSIS (MS).

Preparing and Using: Broad beans are nicest just simmered (after soaking) for about 1 hour, or until they are tender, then drained and liquidised with garlic and seasoning, to make a purée. Serve this with fresh lemon juice and good olive oil, as well as warm bread or freshly cooked EASY FELAFEL (see below) to dip into the earthy-tasting mixture. Sliced tomatoes, spring onions and lettuce go well with it, too. If you add fried onion, garlic and wholewheat breadcrumbs, a broad bean purée can be made into tasty beanburgers and cooked in the same way as felafel.

CHICK PEA *Cicer arietinum*

Neutral

Chick peas have similar qualities to other pulses but they are also notable for their anti-inflammatory action, particularly on the urino-genital system, so they are especially helpful for conditions such as CYSTITIS. They are one of the easier pulses to digest, and one of the most delicious to eat. Their cooking time is variable; it can be about 1 hour but 3 hours is more usual.

Preparing and Using: Try chick peas made into felafel or hummus (see recipes below), simply tossed in garlic butter, or stir-fried with onion, garlic and whole cumin seeds. Chick pea flour, which you can buy at healthfood shops, can be made into fritters and pancakes, as well as being a useful egg replacement for non-dairy recipes. In place of each egg, use 1 tablespoon chick pea flour mixed with enough cold water to form a smooth paste.

EASY FELAFEL

These are very quick to make with a food processor. Serves 4.

> *225 g/8 oz dried chick peas, soaked and cooked*
> *1 small onion, peeled*
> *1 garlic clove, peeled*
> *6–8 good sprigs of parsley*

2 heaped teaspoons ground coriander
sea salt and freshly ground black pepper
100 g/4 oz dried wholewheat crumbs, for coating
oil, for shallow-frying

Drain the chick peas, reserving the liquid. If you are using a food processor, cut the onion into chunks. Put the chunks into the processor with the chick peas, the whole garlic clove, parsley, coriander and seasoning and whizz to a thick purée. Otherwise, mash the chick peas well, grate the onion, crush the garlic, chop the parsley, then mix them together, with the coriander and seasoning. Form into walnut-sized rounds, coat in dried crumbs and shallow-fry or place on an oiled baking sheet and bake at 200°C/400°F/Gas Mark 6 for 30–40 minutes, until browned, turning them over after about 20 minutes, or when the underside is browned. Serve hot, or warm, with a selection of salads and dips.

FAVOURITE HUMMUS

Home-made hummus is nourishing yet light, good for children and convalescents, and soothing if there is inflammation in the urino-genital area. This is a particularly delicious version. It's best to use the very pale tahini made by Cypressa which you can get from Middle Eastern shops. If you can only get the stronger dark type, reduce the amount to 1 teaspoon. Serve hummus as a dip with raw vegetables, spooned over baked potatoes or steamed vegetables, or spread on bread. Serves 2–3.

100 g/4 oz chick peas, soaked and cooked
2 garlic cloves, peeled
2 tablespoons pale tahini
juice of 1 lemon
2 tablespoons olive oil
sea salt and freshly ground black pepper
paprika pepper (optional)

Drain the chick peas, reserving the liquid. Then put the chick peas, garlic, tahini, lemon juice and oil in a food processor and blend thoroughly, until pale and creamy. Add some of the reserved liquid if necessary, to get a light consistency, like softly whipped cream. Season to taste with salt and pepper, spoon into a shallow serving dish and top with a little olive oil, and a sprinkling of paprika pepper if you wish.

141

HARICOT OR CANNELLINI BEAN *Phaseolus vulgaris*

Neutral, diuretic

These white beans have all the qualities of pulses generally and, in addition, are reputed to have particularly good diuretic powers.

Preparing and Using: Haricot beans take 1–1½ hours to cook. They can be made into a delicious salad, with fresh herbs and an oil and vinegar, or oil and lemon, dressing. Mashed, and mixed with fried onions and cumin, basil or coriander, they make good burgers (see EASY FELAFEL, page 140). Or, simmered with onions, garlic and a bay leaf until tender, then whizzed to a purée, they make a soup which is soothing as well as tasty, especially if you snip fresh herbs over the top.

BEANS WITH CORN AND PUMPKIN

This is a soothing and nourishing dish with good diuretic powers. Serves 2.

> 1 *tablespoon olive oil*
> 1 *medium onion, finely chopped*
> 50 *g/2 oz cannellini or haricot beans, soaked and cooked*
> 100 *g/4 oz pumpkin, diced*
> 2 *courgettes, sliced*
> 100 *g/4 oz sweetcorn*
> 2 *tomatoes, skinned and quartered*
> *sea salt and freshly ground black pepper*

Heat the oil in a large pan and fry the onion slowly until it is soft. Add the remaining ingredients, cover and cook gently for about 10 minutes, stirring from time to time, until the vegetables are tender. Add a little water if the mixture begins to stick. Season to taste with salt and pepper, and serve with some hunks of bread, or a baked potato, or just a salad.

LENTIL *Lens esculenta*

Neutral to warming

Both red and brown lentils are warming and rich in protein and iron. They are one of the easiest pulses to digest and one of the quickest to prepare.

Preparing and Using: Red lentils are particularly useful because they cook in only 20 minutes without soaking, although they cook more evenly and quickly, in 10–15 minutes, if left to soak for 1–2 hours before cooking.

It's best to soak brown lentils before cooking; they then take 40–45 minutes. Cooked, drained and mixed with olive oil, slivers of raw onion and lemon juice, brown lentils make a good salad; or they can be added to fried onions and other vegetables, lightly spiced, and served hot.

Both red and brown lentils make good burgers. Cook the brown lentils in the usual way. Red lentils should be cooked, after soaking and draining, in only a little water – 150 ml/5 fl oz to 225–250 g/8–9 oz lentils (dry weight) – to make a thick consistency. Mix with plenty of fried onions and seasoning, then fry or bake as described for EASY FELAFEL (page 140). Red lentils can also be mixed with millet, courgettes and carrots to make a nourishing soup for weak digestions (see recipe on page 158).

QUICK LENTIL AND VEGETABLE CASSEROLE

This is a really nutritious soup or stew which can be made in moments and is good served with hunks of bread or garlic bread. Serves 4.

> 450 g/1 lb frozen or fresh diced root vegetables
> 1 bay leaf
> ½ teaspoon thyme, lemon thyme or savory
> 225 g/8 oz split red lentils
> sea salt and freshly ground black pepper
> lemon juice

Put the root vegetables in a large saucepan with 1 litre/1¾ pints water, the bay leaf, herbs and lentils. Cover, bring to the boil, then cook gently for about 20 minutes until the lentils are tender. Season to taste with salt, pepper and a squeeze of lemon juice.

LENTIL SOUP

Soothing yet strengthening and highly nourishing, this is an excellent food for convalescents or, without the garlic and seasoning, for weaning a vegetarian baby. It can be spiced according to your particular taste and need; the garlic can be left out and cumin seeds, roasted for a moment in a dry pan, can be sprinkled on top; or you could fry 1 teaspoon ground coriander with the onions. Serves 4.

143

1 tablespoon olive oil
2 onions, peeled and chopped
2 carrots, scraped and sliced
255 g/8 oz red lentils
2 garlic cloves, peeled (optional)
sea salt and freshly ground black pepper

Heat the oil in a large saucepan and fry the onions for 5 minutes. Add the carrots, cook for a few seconds, then add the lentils and 1 litre/1¾ pints water. Cover, bring to the boil and simmer for about 20 minutes. Liquidise with the garlic if using. Return the soup to the pan, reheat, and season to taste with salt and pepper.

SPICY LENTIL DAL

Dal is one of the easiest and most useful dishes, and highly nutritious. You can spice it according to your needs; for instance, if you want a more cooling mixture, leave out the ginger and garlic and add plenty of chopped fresh mint and some lemon juice at the end of the cooking time. Serve with steamed brown rice, and SPICED CABBAGE AND CARROTS (page 98) if you wish, or with plain lightly cooked cabbage, and some sliced fresh tomato. Serves 4.

250 g/9 oz red lentils
1 green chilli, halved, deseeded and chopped
2 thick slices of fresh ginger
1 onion, peeled and sliced
½ teaspoon turmeric
1 bay leaf
1–2 large garlic cloves, peeled and crushed (optional)
sea salt

Wash and drain the lentils, then put them in a saucepan with 1 litre/1¾ pints water, the chilli, ginger, onion, turmeric and bay leaf. Cover, bring to the boil, then leave to simmer gently for 30–40 minutes, or until the lentils are very soft. Leave the mixture to stand for about 1 hour if possible. Then remove the onion, bay leaf and ginger. Add the crushed garlic, if using, and season to taste with salt just before serving.

MISO

Neutral to warming, cleansing, tonic

Miso is a paste obtained by fermenting soya beans for 18 months with sea salt, water and a mould called koji. It is one of the very few non-animal products to contain vitamin B12; it is therefore, in Chinese medical terminology, 'strengthening to the blood', and a particularly valuable food for vegans and vegetarians. In Chinese medicine a soup made with miso is rated highly as a winter food, 'warming and tonifying the yang during the yin months of the year'. Some believe that miso can provide protection against radiation, or even get rid of it once it is in the body.

Note: People with KIDNEY PROBLEMS or HYPERTENSION (HIGH BLOOD PRESSURE) should only take miso in moderation because of its high salt content.

Preparing and Using: Four types of miso are available: hacho miso, made from soya beans; genmai miso, made from soya beans and brown rice; mugi miso, made from soya beans and barley; and natto miso, made from soya beans, barley, seaweed and ginger. The lightest and easiest to use is genmai miso.

Transfer the miso from its polythene wrapper to a jar, and store it in the fridge where it will keep for months. When including miso in a soup, always add it towards the end of the cooking time, to preserve the nutrients. You can make a quick soup by dissolving 1 teaspoon miso in a cup of boiling water. Or, for a tastier miso broth, simmer some chopped spring onion, crushed garlic, grated ginger and 1 teaspoon miso in 300 ml/10 fl oz water for 15 minutes. Remove from the heat and season to taste.

MISO, OAT AND VEGETABLE SOUP

A cleansing yet quite substantial vegetable soup. Serves 4.

> 1 *tablespoon olive oil*
> 1 *onion, peeled and chopped*
> 225 *g/8 oz carrots, scrubbed and sliced*
> 3–4 *sticks celery, chopped*
> 50 *g/2 oz rolled oats*
> 1–2 *teaspoons miso*
> *tamari or shoyu*

145

Heat the oil in a large saucepan, then add the onion and fry, with a lid on the pan, for 5 minutes. Put in the carrots and celery, and fry for a further 5 minutes, then add 1 litre/1¾ pints water. Cover, bring to the boil, then simmer gently for about 20 minutes, or until the vegetables are almost tender. Stir in the rolled oats and miso and cook for a further 10–15 minutes. Season with a little tamari or shoyu and serve immediately.

MISO SAUCE

This sauce can be served as an alternative to gravy. It goes particularly well with beanburgers and nut roasts. Serves 4.

> 1 *tablespoon olive oil*
> 2 *teaspoons wholewheat flour*
> 1 *teaspoon miso*
> 1 *tablespoon shoyu or tamari*
> *sea salt*

Heat the oil in a pan and add the flour. Stir over the heat for a few minutes until the flour has browned, then add 150 ml/5 fl oz water and the miso, and stir until thickened. Let the sauce simmer gently for 10 minutes, then add the shoyu or tamari and salt to taste.

MUNG BEAN *Phaseolus aureus*

Very cooling

Mung beans are helpful when there is excessive heat in the body, creating inflammation and redness.

Preparing and Using: Mung beans cook, after soaking, in about 40 minutes. They are also probably the most delicious sprouted bean, and in this form they are an instant food, easy to add to stir-fried vegetable mixtures and salads or to eat as a snack. They can be made into a simple soup as described for haricot and cannellini beans (page 142) – try flavouring the mung bean soup with grated lemon rind or a lemon-flavoured herb such as lemon thyme or, for a more cooling mixture, lemon balm. SPICY LENTIL DAL (see page 144) can also be made with mung beans instead of red lentils.

(DRIED) PEA *Pisum sativum*

Neutral, nutrient, laxative

Dried peas have similar qualities to fresh peas (see page 121), but in a more concentrated form, with useful amounts of protein and B vitamins.

Preparing and Using: Both green and yellow split peas need the usual preliminary soaking, then a slow simmer for 20–30 minutes until tender. They can make an excellent soup, or a purée for serving with other vegetables.

To make a soup, follow the recipe for LENTIL SOUP (page 143) but add some sprigs of mint with the peas and remove these before liquidising. Flavour with a good pinch of ground cloves and snip some fresh mint over the top of each bowl. You can adjust the thickness of this soup to your taste by adding more water.

For a purée, soak, drain and rinse the peas in the usual way. Then put them in a saucepan with cold water to cover (600 ml/1 pint to 225–250 g/8–9 oz peas, dry weight), add a bay leaf and a peeled onion stuck with a few cloves, cover and cook gently for 40–45 minutes, or until the peas are very tender and collapsed. Top up the water level during the cooking time if necessary. Remove the onion, add a knob of butter, and season to taste with sea salt and freshly ground black pepper. An alternative is to fry chopped onion gently in the butter until tender, instead of cooking it whole with the peas; then stir the onion and its buttery juices into the split peas when they are cooked.

RED KIDNEY BEAN *Phaseolus vulgaris*

Neutral to warming, laxative

Like all pulses, red kidney beans are rich in iron and nutrients; they are therefore considered, in Chinese medicine, to be particularly 'nourishing to the blood' and helpful for ANAEMIA. They are certainly one of the tastiest pulses and have probably the best laxative action to ease CONSTIPATION.

Preparing and Using: Red kidney beans are the ones which you need to be particularly careful about boiling for at least 10 minutes, after soaking, to eliminate any possible toxicity. After this you can let them simmer gently until tender (about 1¼ hours of cooking in all). Cooked red kidney beans can be added to any vegetable casserole or stir-fry.

One of the simplest ways of serving them is to add about 225–275 g/8–10 oz cooked drained beans to an onion which you have softened in a little oil or butter, with, if you like, a crushed garlic clove and a chopped chilli. Mash the beans roughly, to give a chunky texture, then add 1–2 skinned, chopped tomatoes and seasoning. Stir over the heat until warmed through. This is good with fresh coriander snipped over the top, served with slices of ripe avocado and some tortilla chips.

RED BEAN CHILLI WITH CUMIN AND FRESH CORIANDER

This mixture is good hot, served with brown rice or baked potatoes; or it can be used to fill tacos, or served cold, as a salad. Serves 4.

2 tablespoons olive oil
1 onion, peeled and chopped
1 large garlic clove, peeled and crushed
1 green chilli, deseeded and sliced
1 large red pepper, deseeded and chopped
175 g/6 oz red kidney beans, soaked and cooked
6 tomatoes, skinned and quartered
1 tablespoon tomato purée
1 teaspoon ground cumin
sea salt and freshly ground black pepper
Barbados sugar
1–2 tablespoons chopped fresh coriander (if available)

Heat the oil in a large saucepan, add the onion and cook, covered, for 5 minutes. Then add the garlic, chilli and pepper and cook for a further 5 minutes. Now put in the beans, tomatoes, tomato purée, cumin and 300 ml/10 fl oz water. Bring to the boil, then simmer gently for 15–20 minutes, until all the vegetables are tender and the liquid has reduced to a sauce-like consistency. Season to taste with salt and pepper and sugar. Serve sprinkled with chopped fresh coriander if available.

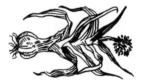

SOYA BEANS *Glycine max*

Neutral to cooling

These have similar properties to tofu (see below) but are not as versatile or easy to prepare and eat. Both soya flour and soya milk share these qualities.

Preparing and Using: Soak soya beans overnight; drain and rinse them. Cover with plenty of water, boil hard for 10 minutes, then cook for about 4 hours or until tender. They are best in strongly flavoured dishes. Soya flour is widely available and can be added to recipes to enrich them when extra protein is needed, or it can be used as an egg replacement, as described for chick pea flour (page 140).

TOFU

Neutral to cooling

Tofu, sometimes called beancurd, is very cooling and has similar properties to mung beans (page 146). Being quite moist as well, it is helpful for dryness anywhere in the body. Tofu is valuable as a non-dairy source of calcium, and, unlike dairy sources, it contains iron too.

Preparing and Using: Delicious fresh tofu can be bought from Chinese shops and some healthfood shops. Stored in cold water in the fridge, it will keep for 2–3 days. Tofu is also available in vacuum packs, in varying degrees of firmness. The firm type is most useful for savoury dishes, stir-fries and vegetable mixtures, whilst the softer, 'silken' type is best for making dips; combining with herbs, olive oil, lemon juice or wine vinegar to make dressings; or whizzing with a little honey or apple juice concentrate into creamy toppings or purées with fruit. See TOFU APRICOT FOOL (page 178) and STRAWBERRY AND TOFU WHIZZ (page 202). With any type of packaged tofu, drain off the liquid before using unless the recipe says otherwise. Packaged tofu freezes well.

GINGER-MARINATED TOFU

This and the following recipe are both excellent quick savoury dishes and can be eaten hot or cold. Serve them with cooked vegetables or salad and brown rice or millet. Serves 2.

2 tablespoons tamari or shoyu
1 garlic clove, peeled and crushed
2–3 teaspoons grated fresh ginger
1 block of firm tofu, drained and sliced

Mix the tamari or shoyu in a bowl with the garlic and ginger. Add the tofu, mix gently, then leave to marinate for 20–30 minutes, or longer if possible, stirring from time to time. To serve, heat through in a covered casserole in a moderate oven; or on a plate over a pan of steaming water. This is good sprinkled with some GOMASIO, or sesame salt (see page 172).

LIME-MARINATED TOFU WITH CHILLI AND BLACK PEPPER

Serves 2.

rind and juice of 1 well-scrubbed unwaxed lime
1 dried red chilli
1 teaspoon black peppercorns, crushed
1 tablespoon olive oil
1 tablespoon tamari or shoyu
1 block of firm tofu, drained and sliced
sea salt

Mix the lime rind and juice, chilli, black pepper, oil and tamari or shoyu in a bowl. Add the tofu and stir gently, then leave to marinate for at least 30 minutes, stirring occasionally. Season to taste with a little salt, heat, and serve as described in the recipe above.

STIR-FRIED TOFU WITH CARROTS AND ONIONS

This is a light main course dish, rich in protein. Herbs or spices can be added according to specific tastes and needs; aniseed or fennel seeds can be fried with the onion and carrot, and a variety of chopped fresh herbs can be added at the end. Serve it with some brown rice and some shoyu soy sauce to sprinkle over. Serves 2 (or 4 with other dishes).

1 block of firm tofu, drained
2 carrots
2 onions
1 tablespoon olive oil
chopped fresh coriander, parsley or other fresh herbs (optional)

150

Dice the tofu; scrape and slice the carrots; peel and slice the onions. Heat the oil in a large saucepan, frying pan or wok and add the carrots and onions. Stir-fry for about 5 minutes, until the vegetables are softening, then add the tofu, and stir-fry for another few minutes, until the tofu has heated through.

See also PUMPKIN AND TOFU PURÉE (page 125).

Grains

Grains have an important role to play in helping us counteract illness and stay well. As the World Health Organisation has pointed out, in the healthiest diets at least 50 per cent of the day's calorie intake comes from grains. This proportion is similar to that which has been advised in traditional Chinese medicine for thousands of years.

A good way of planning a healthy meal is to start with a grain, or with potatoes (which, being starchy, can be classified with grains for this purpose), then add vegetables, aiming to eat at least 450 g/1 lb of vegetables and fruit each day. You should also include pulses, with small quantities of meat, fish and dairy produce as a flavouring and garnish if you wish.

Simply cooked grains are very versatile: they go with numerous vegetables; can be flavoured in many ways with different herbs and spices; can be served hot or cold; and go with every meal of the day. In terms of Chinese medicine, grains are mainly neutral in heat, so they can be warmed up with hot herbs and spices such as garlic, ginger, basil and thyme, or cooled by adding mint, parsley, artichokes or cucumber, depending on your condition and how you are feeling.

It may take a while to get used to the flavour of some of the more unusual grains so you may prefer to cook them with brown rice. Wheat grains, millet, pot barley, groats and rye can all be cooked in this way, replacing ¼–½ of the rice with them, and cooking in the usual way.

BUYING AND STORING

Grains can be bought in different forms: whole grains; flaked, or whole grains which have been rolled and flattened; as flour, and, in some cases, products such as bread and pasta. Wholewheat flour, bread and pasta are widely available, as are rolled oats, brown rice and oatmeal. For the other grains and flours you will probably have to go to a healthfood or wholefood shop, where you should find a good selection. Buy in small quantities and store in jars or tins in a cool, dry place.

151

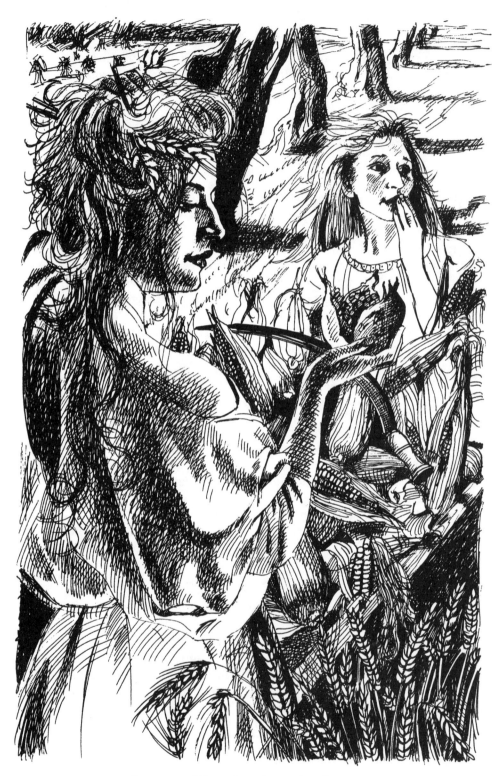

Demeter and Persephone harvesting the corn

COOKING

Grains are really easy to cook and, with the exception of maize (see page 155), the basic method is the same for all of them. Put the grain in a heavy-based saucepan with double its volume in cold water (that is, 1 cup grain to 2 cups water, or 225 g/8 oz grain to 600 ml/1 pint water). Bring to the boil, then cover and cook over the lowest heat until the grain is tender and all the water absorbed. This takes 20 minutes for millet and buckwheat, and 45 minutes for the others. Wholewheat grains can take longer and benefit from 1–1½ hours soaking in cold water first (see page 164).

A variation, using buckwheat, millet or rice, is to roast the grain, either in a dry saucepan, or in 1 tablespoon oil or butter, stirring over a moderate heat for 1–2 minutes until the grain begins to smell roasted and, in the case of millet, to pop. Then add the water. You can sauté garlic, ginger, spices, onion and other vegetables with the oil or butter for a few minutes, before adding the grain, for added flavour and interest.

Serving cooked grains cold, as a salad, adds variety and is more cooling in hot weather, or if you have a hot condition. Almost any cooked or suitably chopped or grated raw vegetables, chopped fresh herbs, nuts and seeds can be mixed with the grains and dressed with 1–2 tablespoons olive oil and some fresh lemon juice to make a salad.

BARLEY *Hordeum vulgare*

Cooling, tonic, anti-inflammatory, diuretic

Barley has a cooling, anti-inflammatory and anti-spasmodic action on the digestive system, helping acidity, stomach burning, HAEMORRHOIDS (PILES), ULCERATIVE COLITIS, DIVERTICULITIS and similar problems. Like brown rice and millet, barley has an important regulatory action on the intestines, improving both DIARRHOEA and CONSTIPATION. It is also well-known for its anti-inflammatory action on the genito-urinary tract, useful in complaints such as CYSTITIS and NEPHRITIS.

Preparing and Using: Unrefined barley, known as 'pot barley', should not be confused with pearl barley, the type found in most shops, which has had some of its outer layers removed. Despite appearances, pot barley, which you can get at healthfood shops, is quite soft and pale

153

when cooked and easy to eat when mixed with brown rice (as described on page 151).

To make barley water, a soothing, cooling drink which is helpful for CYSTITIS, NEPHRITIS and spasmodic digestive problems, simmer 50 g/2 oz barley in 1 litre/1¾ pints water for 40 minutes. Cool, strain and add a little fresh lemon juice if liked. Drink over 24 hours.

BARLEY, POTATO AND CABBAGE SOUP

A nourishing soup to clear inflammation and help digestion. Serves 4.

>*50 g/2 oz pot barley*
>*1 potato, scrubbed or peeled and diced*
>*50 g/2 oz cabbage, shredded*
>*½ teaspoon aniseed (optional)*
>*sea salt and freshly ground black pepper*

Put the barley in a large saucepan with 1 litre/1¾ pints water and boil for 25 minutes. Then add the potato and simmer for a further 10 minutes, until the potato is almost cooked. Finally, put in the cabbage and aniseed, if using, and cook for about 5 minutes more, until the cabbage is tender. Season to taste with salt and pepper, and serve.

BUCKWHEAT *Polygonum fagopyrum*

Neutral, circulatory, tonic

Botanically speaking, buckwheat is a seed rather than a grain, although it is usually grouped with grains and shares many of their attributes. Buckwheat has a balancing action on the intestines, helping both DIARRHOEA and CONSTIPATION. It is rich in minerals and vitamins but its most notable component is rutin, which makes it an important food for all CIRCULATORY PROBLEMS, including VARICOSE VEINS and BROKEN CAPILLARIES. Some authorities believe that it can improve HYPERTENSION (HIGH BLOOD PRESSURE). Cooked buckwheat, also known as kasha, is a popular dish in Poland and Russia, especially during the winter months.

Preparing and Using: Buckwheat can be bought roasted and unroasted; roasting makes it more warming and tonifying, as well as improving the flavour. Buckwheat flour and pasta are also available; try making pancakes or scones using half wheat flour and half buckwheat flour.

Some people love buckwheat, others find it difficult to get used to the taste. Like any grain, it is much improved by the addition of some butter, stirred in after cooking, and perhaps a little crushed garlic. Some fried onion or mushrooms are a good addition, too. It's good served as an accompaniment to robust vegetables such as beetroot – try it with the HEARTY BEETROOT SOUP (page 93) or with carrots, parsnips, celery or leeks. Or try the soup below.

BUCKWHEAT WINTER SOUP

To increase the circulation and warm the body. Serves 4.

> 1 *tablespoon olive oil*
> 2 *onions, peeled and chopped*
> 225 *g/8 oz carrots, scrubbed and chopped*
> 2 *garlic cloves, peeled and crushed*
> 2–3 *teaspoons freshly grated ginger*
> 100 *g/4 oz roasted buckwheat*
> *sea salt and freshly ground black pepper*

Heat the oil in a large saucepan; add the onions and carrots and sauté gently, with a lid on the pan, for 10 minutes. Add the garlic, ginger and buckwheat and stir-fry for a further 1–2 minutes, then pour in 1 litre/ 1¾ pints water. Cover, bring to the boil, then cook gently for about 20 minutes, until the buckwheat and vegetables are cooked.

MAIZE (SWEETCORN) *Zea mays*

Neutral, tonic, diuretic

Nourishing and slightly tonic, corn is an easy food to eat because of its versatility. It can be eaten on or off the cob, as grains and as flour (polenta), and it always tastes delicious. In many ancient texts corn is said to be a good tonic for the heart, a quality confirmed by recent research. Corn – especially the silk wrapped around the cobs (see below) – is also a good diuretic and kidney-cleanser, valuable for KIDNEY INFLAMMATION, CYSTITIS and OBESITY.

Preparing and Using: Maize is available on the cob, both fresh and frozen; frozen off the cob, as sweetcorn; dried, as 'popping corn'; and dried and ground, as polenta.

To prepare fresh sweetcorn, remove the leaves and silky threads and trim off the stalk. Immerse in a large panful of boiling unsalted water and simmer for about 10 minutes, until the kernels are tender. Don't overcook, or they toughen. Drain and serve with melted butter, and a little sea salt and freshly ground black pepper if you wish.

To cook just the kernels, cut these from the cob, then cook in boiling water for 2–5 minutes. A single cob produces about 75 g/3 oz sweetcorn kernels.

For cornsilk tea, infuse the threads from a cob of corn in a cupful of boiling water for 5–10 minutes, strain and serve.

CORN, LEEK AND LENTIL SOUP

This soup is light yet filling. It's helpful for CYSTITIS, KIDNEY INFLAMMATION, and also, with its diuretic properties, for OBESITY. Serves 4.

> *50 g/2 oz split red lentils*
> *2 leeks, washed and sliced*
> *100 g/4 oz sweetcorn, frozen or cut from a cob*
> *juice of ½ lemon*
> *sea salt and freshly ground black pepper*
> *chopped fresh parsley*

Put the lentils in a saucepan with 600 ml/1 pint water. Boil for 10 minutes, then add the leeks and simmer gently for another 15 minutes, or until the lentils and leeks are soft. Add the sweetcorn and cook for a further 5 minutes, until the corn is tender. Add the lemon juice, season to taste with salt and pepper, sprinkle over some chopped fresh parsley, and serve.

POLENTA

Serves 4.

> *225 g/8 oz polenta*
> *2 heaped tablespoons chopped fresh parsley*
> *6 spring onions, chopped*
> *sea salt*

Put the polenta in a pan with 1 litre/1¾ pints water. Bring to the boil, then turn down the heat. Simmer gently for 30 minutes, stirring often with a wooden spoon. At the end of the cooking time, stir in the chopped parsley and spring onions. Mix well, taste, and add salt if necessary. Oil a deepish mould, pour in the polenta, and allow it to cool before turning out. Cut in slices, warm through in a covered dish in the oven and serve with a fresh tomato sauce and green vegetable; or fry the slices in oil, and serve with a green salad. This, too, is good with a fresh tomato sauce.

HONEY POPCORN

This is a healthy snack for children.

> *corn or sunflower oil*
> *popping corn*
> 6 *tablespoons clear honey*
> 15 *g/½ oz butter*

Put enough oil into a heavy-based saucepan to cover the bottom. Add enough popping corn to cover the bottom lightly, allowing a little space between kernels. Put a lid on the saucepan and place over a high heat. Shake the pan often to prevent the bottom from burning. You will hear the kernels popping inside. When the popping has stopped, remove from the heat. Put the honey in a large saucepan with the butter, bring to the boil and boil for 3 minutes. Remove from the heat and add the popcorn. Mix quickly so that all the corn is coated with the honey, allow to cool a little, and serve.

MILLET *Milium effusum; Panicum milliaceum*

Cooling, tonic, soothing

This healing, soothing grain, rich in minerals and vitamins, with a delicious, sweet flavour, deserves to be more widely known and used. Like rice and barley, millet has a cooling and soothing action on the digestive system, helping acidity, stomach burning, PILES, ULCERATIVE COLITIS, DIVERTICULITIS and similar complaints, as well as regulating the action of the intestines, helping both DIARRHOEA and CONSTIPATION. In Europe millet, if eaten regularly at least 3 times a week, is renowned as a strengthener of the nails and hair. It may therefore be helpful in counteracting HAIR LOSS.

Preparing and Using: Millet can be bought in the form of whole grains, flaked, and as flour. Once you get accustomed to the flavour, it can become as useful a basic as brown rice. One advantage of millet is

157

that it cooks quickly, in 20 minutes. In this, it makes a good partner for red lentils, which also cook fast; together they are highly nutritious.

MILLET, LENTIL, COURGETTE AND CARROT SOUP

A simple nourishing soup for delicate digestions. Serves 4.

> *100 g/4 oz split red lentils*
> *100 g/4 oz millet*
> *225 g/8 oz carrots, scrubbed and sliced*
> *225 g/8 oz courgettes, sliced*
> *sea salt and freshly ground black pepper*

Cover the lentils with cold water and soak for 30–60 minutes. Then drain, rinse and put them in a saucepan with the millet, carrots and 1 litre/1¾ pints water. Cover, bring to the boil, then simmer gently for about 10 minutes, or until the lentils and millet are almost soft. Add the courgettes and cook for a further 3–5 minutes, until the courgettes are tender. Season to taste with salt and pepper.

MULTICOLOUR MILLET SALAD

A good recipe for general vitality, and, like all millet recipes, particularly good for the hair. Serves 4.

> *225 g/8 oz millet*
> *1 large carrot, scrubbed and sliced*
> *4 tomatoes, sliced*
> *a 5 cm/2 in piece of cucumber, sliced*
> *1 red pepper, deseeded and chopped*
> *1 avocado, peeled and sliced*
> *fresh basil leaves, torn or roughly chopped*
> *juice of 1 lemon*
> *2–4 tablespoons olive oil*
> *sea salt and freshly ground black pepper*

Put the millet in a dry pan and stir over the heat for a minute or so until it smells toasted and the grains begin to pop. Standing well back, pour in 400 ml/14 fl oz water. Allow the mixture to come up to the boil, then cover and cook over a gentle heat for 20 minutes, until the millet is tender and all the water absorbed. Allow to cool, then add all the remaining ingredients, forking them gently through the millet.

158

OATS *Avena sativa*

Warming, tonic, beneficial to the nerves

Rich in vitamins and minerals, warming and tonic, oats have the ability to raise the energy and general vitality. They are helpful for children and convalescents, as well as being a traditional breakfast food in many cold countries.

Oats are one of the best tonics for the nervous system, useful for people who are exhausted through NERVOUS TENSION and STRESS. Many herbalists and homeopaths prescribe tincture of oats – 10–20 drops in water – to restore weak and frail nerves.

Tests have shown that supplementing a normal diet with oat bran, or eating a bowl of porridge for breakfast and including oats in 2 other meals during the day can lower blood cholesterol by an average of 20 per cent. Oats – and especially oat bran – are highly recommended for people with sugar problems such as DIABETES and HYPOGLYCAEMIA, because their soluble fibre content can slow the rate of sugar metabolism, thus relieving strain on the pancreas.

Oats contain phosphorus, which can be helpful for memory; and, according to Dr Valnet, they stimulate the thyroid gland and are therefore useful for HYPOTHYROIDISM. Those with HYPERTHYROIDISM can also take oats but should do so in moderation, perhaps once or twice a week.

Some sources attribute aphrodisiac properties to oats, and the ability to increase fertility; during lactation they help to increase the supply of milk.

Preparing and Using: Whole oat grains, called 'groats', can be bought from healthfood shops, as can oat bran and coarse, medium or fine oatmeal, and 'jumbo oats', which are flattened oat grains. Rolled oats, or 'porridge oats', as they are sometimes called, are widely available. Groats can be cooked with brown rice as described for several other grains (see page 151); jumbo oats can be made into porridge and biscuits; whilst oatmeal, particularly medium ground, is useful for making porridge and oatcakes and for thickening soups. Oats do not keep well; buy in small quantities and do not use them if they smell at all rancid.

PORRIDGE

Quick and easy to make, porridge is one of the healthiest and most warming breakfasts you can have; it also makes a soothing light supper dish. Cooking raisins in the mixture gives natural sweetness; alternatively you can add to this by topping the cooked porridge with sliced banana, reduced-sugar preserves, real maple syrup, clear honey or Barbados sugar, and a little milk or soya milk, cream, or ALMOND CREAM (see page 167). You can make the porridge even more warming, and add an interesting flavour, by sprinkling the top with some ground ginger, cinnamon or grated nutmeg. Alternatively, eat the porridge plain, in true Scottish style, with just a sprinkling of sea salt! Serves 1.

50 g/2 oz medium oatmeal or porridge oats
40 g/1½ oz raisins (optional)

Bring 600 ml/1 pint water to the boil in a medium-sized saucepan. Gradually stir in the oatmeal or porridge oats, and add the raisins if using. Continue to stir for about 3 minutes, as the mixture comes back to the boil and thickens. Remove from the heat and leave to stand for a few minutes; the porridge will get thicker as it cools.

OATCAKES

Good for NERVOUS TENSION and STRESS, these are a tasty alternative to wheat products and crispbreads. They are excellent spread with unsalted butter, honey and a sprinkling of cinnamon, or the indulgent AVOCADO, BANANA, CAROB AND HONEY SPREAD on page 180. Makes 20–24.

175 g/6 oz medium oatmeal
½ teaspoon salt
15 g/½ oz butter or margarine
extra oatmeal for rolling

Put the oatmeal in a bowl with the salt and the butter or margarine and pour in 150 ml/5 fl oz boiling water. Mix to a sticky dough. Leave for 5 minutes, to allow the oatmeal to expand and the dough to become manageable, then turn out on to a surface sprinkled with oatmeal and knead lightly. Roll the mixture out as thinly as you can (it's probably easiest to do this in 2 batches), sprinkling with extra oatmeal to prevent sticking. Cut into circles using a large round pastry cutter and put close together on a baking sheet. Bake for 15–20 minutes, until dry and crisp but not browned. Cool on a wire rack.

SAVOURY CRUMBLE TOPPING

This topping – which, like oatcakes, is good for the nervous system – can be used to turn many vegetable mixtures into a main course; try it on the BUTTERED CELERY on page 103. It is best on moist vegetable mixtures, as the oats absorb some of the liquid: add a little vegetable water if necessary. For a sweet version, good on top of stewed apples, pears or plums, replace the thyme and salt with 1 tablespoon Barbados sugar. Makes enough to top a medium-sized gratin, serving 4.

> 100 g/4 oz jumbo oats
> 1 tablespoon light olive oil or tasteless vegetable oil
> 50 g/2 oz flaked almonds
> ½ teaspoon thyme
> sea salt

Set the oven to 180°C/350°F/Gas Mark 4. Put the oats and oil in a bowl and mix together until the oats are all coated with the oil. Then add the almonds, thyme, and salt to taste. Put your chosen vegetable in a shallow heatproof dish and spoon the oat crumble on top. Bake for 20–30 minutes, until crisp and lightly browned.

BROWN RICE *Oryza sativa*

Neutral, harmonising

Brown rice – which is rice in its whole state, without the vitamin-rich outer layers removed – works in a harmonising and nourishing way on the digestive system and throughout the body. As a neutral and strengthening food, brown rice is recommended for imbalances of both yin and yang.

Because of its high vitamin and mineral content, brown rice nourishes the body whilst at the same time gently soothing the nervous system. It removes inflammation and spasms from the digestive system and is thus valuable for INDIGESTION, ABDOMINAL SWELLING, ULCERS, COLIC and DIVERTICULITIS.

Brown rice also has a good harmonising action on the intestines, making it helpful for mild cases of DIARRHOEA and for CONSTIPATION. In addition, the fact that it has up to 7 layers of bran makes brown rice a rich source of fibre and thus of great value in keeping the intestines healthy.

BROWN RICE WATER can be made as described for BARLEY WATER on

161

page 154, or by boiling brown rice with an extra cupful of water (3–4 cups water to 1 cup of rice) and pouring off the extra water when the rice is cooked. This is helpful not only for digestive problems but for inflammation anywhere in the body, including the respiratory and urinary systems.

Preparing and Using: Long-grain brown rice, the most useful for general cookery, is widely available. Brown Basmati rice, with fine, slim, pointed grains, and round or medium-grain rice, as well as brown rice flour, are available from healthfood shops. Brown rice, cooked as described on page 153, goes well with virtually all vegetables and also makes an excellent base for other flavourings. So if you need to take a particular herb or spice, adding it to brown rice is a good way of doing so.

Leftover brown rice can be made into a delicious salad: fried in 1 tablespoon oil with other vegetables and herbs and spices to taste, or mixed with chopped walnuts, and perhaps fried onions and garlic, and used to stuff large tomatoes; parboiled, scooped-out courgettes; pieces of squash or peppers of any colour; or baked, halved, scooped-out aubergines – the scooped-out flesh can be added to the mixture, too.

Another good mixture is WALNUT RICE; to make this you cook walnut halves or pieces with brown rice, allowing 50 g/2 oz rice, 15–25 g/½–1 oz walnuts and 150 ml/5 fl oz water per serving. Some lightly fried onion and crushed garlic can be added to the cooked rice, perhaps a few fried mushrooms, and any chopped herbs you fancy. This is good on its own, or, like leftover rice, it can be used as a stuffing for vegetables.

SPICED RICE

A warming, fragrant rice to serve with mixed vegetables and SPICY LENTIL DAL (page 144). Serves 4.

> 225 g/8 oz brown rice (preferably Basmati)
> 25 g/1 oz butter
> 6 black peppercorns
> 3 cloves
> 4–5 cardamom pods, lightly crushed with a teaspoon or rolling pin
> ⅓ cinnamon stick
> ½ teaspoon turmeric
> 1 bay leaf
> 1 teaspoon salt

Put the rice in a sieve and wash under the cold tap until the water runs clear. Shake the sieve well to get rid of as much water as possible, then leave on one side to drain. Heat the butter in a medium-sized heavy-based saucepan and add the rice and all the spices. Stir over the heat for 2–3 minutes, until the spices smell aromatic and the rice starts to look opaque. Then add 600 ml/1 pint water and the salt. Bring to the boil, cover, reduce the heat, and leave to cook gently for 45 minutes.

RYE *Seacale cereale*

Neutral, circulatory, anti-diabetic

Rye contains rutin and so helps CIRCULATORY PROBLEMS in a similar way to buckwheat, although the effect of rye is not as pronounced. Dr Valnet considers that, again like buckwheat, rye can make the blood more fluid and thus help prevent the formation of clots. He maintains that illnesses associated with clogged arteries are less common in countries which have a high consumption of rye. Rye can also be useful as part of a general programme for lowering HIGH BLOOD PRESSURE. Like oats, rye can be helpful for DIABETES and sugar problems such as HYPOGLYCAEMIA.

Preparing and Using: You can get whole rye grains and brown rye flour from healthfood shops and rye bread is available from many supermarkets. If you do not find rye palatable on its own, try cooking some whole rye grains with brown rice, as suggested on page 151, or adding a proportion of rye flour to an easy home-made bread mix.

WHEAT *Triticum vulgare*

Slightly cooling, tonic

Wholewheat, like most other whole grains, contains many minerals and vitamins and is a very nourishing source of energy, whereas refined wheat – and other refined cereals – supply calories without giving much true nourishment. It is therefore important to choose wholewheat bread and pasta, preferably made from organically grown flours, in preference to the white, refined varieties. Wheatgerm, the heart of the wheat, which is removed during the milling of white flour, can be bought from healthfood shops and is rich in minerals and vitamins. It is useful for sprinkling over foods and drinks when extra nourishment is required.

Like barley and millet, wheat cools the blood and helps to prevent inflammation, especially when cooked whole. For this purpose you can cook wholewheat grains with another grain such as brown rice. Whole, unrefined and uncrushed grains are also reputed to strengthen the heart and kidneys.

Wheat is thought to have a mildly harmonising action on the nervous system, boosting it when weak and calming it when over-active.

Note: Wheat should not be taken by people who are allergic to gluten, such as those suffering from COELIAC DISEASE.

Preparing and Using: Most healthfood shops stock wholewheat grains, as well as a range of products made from them: wholewheat flour, wheatgerm, bran, bread and pasta. Cook the wheat grains as described on page 153; they can be soaked first in their cooking liquid to reduce the cooking time if you wish. They are quite chewy, but good mixed in equal parts with brown rice.

Another method is to soak them for at least 1 hour, boil them for 10–15 minutes, then transfer them to a lidded casserole or covered bowl and cook them in the top of a steamer for 1–2 hours, or until the grains have burst and are tender. They can then be mixed with dried fruits and warming spices (such as cinnamon and ginger), and perhaps some milk, cream or nut milk. This makes a dish resembling the old English frumenty – good for breakfast or a light meal. Or you could mix the cooked wheat with cooked vegetables to make a main course; alternatively combine the cooked grains with a good olive oil and lemon dressing, some grated carrot, sliced onions and crushed garlic, for a chewy but interesting and tasty salad.

Bulgur wheat, a cracked and precooked grain, is also widely available at healthfood shops, supermarkets and Middle Eastern shops. This grain is not as wholesome as the wholewheat grains, although it is pleasant for a change and quick to prepare. Try it in TABBOULEH salad (page 74); or serve it hot by tossing 250 g/9 oz grains in 25 g/1 oz melted butter or oil in a pan, then adding 600 ml/1 pint boiling water, covering and cooking for 10 minutes, until all the water has been absorbed and the grains are separate.

WHEAT, CARROT AND CELERIAC SOUP

This is a main course soup, good for the nervous system. It's easy to make but you'll need to allow time for the wheat to soak beforehand. Serves 4.

> *175 g/6 oz wholewheat grains*
> *2 tablespoons olive oil*
> *1 onion, peeled and chopped*
> *225 g/8 oz carrots, scrubbed and sliced*
> *225 g/8 oz celeriac, peeled and diced*
> *sea salt and freshly ground black pepper*
> *chopped fresh parsley*

Put the wheat grains in a saucepan with 1.2 litres/2 pints water, cover, bring to the boil, then leave to soak for at least 1 hour (preferably longer, even overnight). Heat the oil in another saucepan and fry the onion for 5 minutes; then add the carrots and celeriac and fry for a further 5 minutes. Add the wheat grains and their soaking liquid. Cover, bring to the boil, then simmer gently for about 1¼ hours (or 25 minutes in a pressure cooker), until the wheat is tender and the grains have burst open. Season to taste with salt and pepper, sprinkle with chopped fresh parsley, and serve.

Nuts and Seeds

Nuts and seeds are concentrated sources of many vitamins, minerals and oils. They add richness and interest to dishes, and, although they are expensive, they are only needed in small quantities. They are easy to eat and use and are one of the healthiest 'convenience foods', valuable for people who are using a great deal of energy or who need to build up their strength.

BUYING, STORING AND USING

As they contain a high proportion of oils, nuts and seeds can become rancid if kept for too long. Always buy them in small quantities from a reliable source and either store in jars or tins in a cool dry place, or in the fridge or freezer. The same principles apply to nut oils: buy good-quality cold-pressed oils in small quantities and keep them in the fridge.

Just a few nuts or seeds sprinkled over cooked grains, vegetables, salads or fruits greatly increase their food value and can turn a simple

165

dish into a main course. Nuts can be ground and made into sweet or savoury dishes. Added to water and heated gently, they make a nourishing non-starch thickener for sauces. Or they can be whizzed, with water, into thick creams or milks and used as drinks or toppings for both sweet and savoury dishes.

ALMOND *Prunus amygdalus var. dulcis*

Neutral, tonic

Sweet almonds have many medicinal and healing properties. They can be used whole or ground, as a flour and a milk. Almond oil is also valuable.

Whole and ground almonds are well known for their rich vitamin and mineral content. They contain a high proportion of potassium phosphate, a 'brain' food; calcium phosphate, a 'bone' food; and magnesium phosphate, a 'flesh' food. Almonds are therefore a particularly valuable food at times of rapid growth, during convalescence, in old age and during physical and mental activity. They are reputed to greatly strengthen the nervous system, improve the memory, build up the strength generally and increase sexual vigour. Almonds in all forms make a good tonic for the respiratory system, recommended for those who have weak and dry lungs with a tendency to COLDS, COUGHS and BRONCHITIS.

A milk made from almonds (see below) makes an excellent substitute for cow's or goat's milk. Being anti-inflammatory and anti-spasmodic, it is useful during convalescence when extra nourishment is needed but the digestion may be weak. It can also soothe the genito-urinary and respiratory systems.

The healing properties of oil of sweet almonds have been appreciated throughout the centuries. It makes an excellent massage oil, toning and rejuvenating, especially when there is DRY, SCALY SKIN.

Taken internally, almond oil can have a soothing laxative action, helping CONSTIPATION and digestion in general. Start by taking 1 teaspoon (½ teaspoon for children unless they are under 15 months), gradually doubling the amount if required.

Preparing and Using: Almonds are widely available – whole, blanched, flaked or ground – and edible almond oil can be bought from healthfood shops. Try eating 10–12 almonds a day, or 1–2 tablespoons ground almonds. You could sprinkle these over a salad of fresh or cooked fruit; or have them for breakfast, with rolled oats, honey and a sprinkling of cinnamon. They can be mixed with a tiny bit of honey (just enough to make them hold together) and a dash of real almond essence or orange flower water, to make a healthy almond paste. Ground almonds also make a particularly good milk and a soothing, nourishing jelly.

ALMOND MILK

Makes 300–400 ml/10–15 fl oz.

50 g/2 oz whole almonds

Put the almonds in a small saucepan and cover with 200–300 ml/7–10 fl oz water. Bring to the boil and boil for 1 minute. Remove from the heat and allow to cool slightly, then pop the almonds out of their skins. Put the skinned almonds in a liquidiser or food processor with the water and whizz until smooth.

ALMOND CREAM

Makes 250–300 ml/8–10 fl oz.

100 g/4 oz whole almonds
vanilla pod or real vanilla essence (optional)
clear honey (optional)

Blanch the almonds by bringing them to the boil in 150 ml/5 fl oz water, as described for ALMOND MILK (see above), then whizz them to a purée in a food processor or liquidiser with the water. A small piece of vanilla pod or a few drops of real vanilla essence can be added to the nuts before liquidising. Sweeten with a dash of honey if you wish.

SWEET ALMOND JELLY

A good dish for invalids, babies and anyone who wants something that is nourishing yet light and easy to digest. Serves 4.

100 g/4 oz ground almonds
2 teaspoons gelozone (vegetable jelling agent)
2–4 tablespoons apple juice concentrate or clear honey
a few drops of real almond essence
a few flaked almonds or chopped preserved ginger to decorate
    (optional)

Put the ground almonds and gelozone in a saucepan. Measure 600 ml/
1 pint water and add a little to the almonds and gelozone to make a
paste, stirring until it is smooth. Gradually add the rest of the water.
Then put the pan over a gentle heat and bring to the boil, stirring often.
Remove from the heat and add the apple juice concentrate or clear
honey and the almond essence. Pour the mixture into 4 individual
dishes, leave to cool and set. Decorate with a few flaked almonds or
some chopped ginger, if you wish, before serving.

CHESTNUT *Castanea sativa*

Warming, nourishing

Although usually classified with nuts, the chestnut contains more starch
and less oil than other nuts, and is therefore more like a grain in its
composition. It mildly strengthens the yang energy and nourishes the
muscles, and is also reputed to improve the nervous system. It contains
useful amounts of calcium, magnesium, phosphorus, iron and B
vitamins and is particularly good in the winter months, especially if you
are engaged in physical work outside or are feeling cold and weak.

Note: People with a weak and SLOW DIGESTION should consume
chestnuts only in moderation.

Preparing and Using: Chestnuts can be bought fresh in autumn and
winter, and dried chestnuts and chestnut flour can be bought all the
year round. Dried chestnuts are particularly convenient because the
fiddly task of removing the hard brown skin has already been done; they
just need soaking and cooking. Soak them for a few hours, or alternatively, you can bring them to the boil, leave them to soak for 1 hour,
then simmer them for 1–2 hours, until tender.

   If you buy fresh chestnuts, make a cut in the skin, then boil them for a
few minutes until the cut opens and the skin can be removed with the
aid of a sharp knife. The chestnuts then need to be simmered in water for
about 15 minutes, or until tender.

   Once cooked, both dried and fresh chestnuts make a delicious addition to vegetable stews, casseroles and stir-fries; their affinity with
Brussels sprouts is well-known and they are also delicious added to
cooked cabbage, or cooked slowly with red cabbage.

   Try a mixture of lightly fried sliced onions, mushrooms and chestnuts;
or mash cooked chestnuts and add onions and garlic cooked in butter,

and some seasoning. This mixture can be used as a stuffing: it's excellent rolled up in cabbage leaves which have been dipped in boiling water to soften. Pack the stuffed leaves closely together in a casserole or shallow pan, pour some water or stock around them, dot with butter, cover and cook very gently on top of the stove, or in the oven, until the cabbage leaves are very tender. Serve with mashed or baked potatoes and MISO SAUCE (page 146). Or try mixing cooked chestnuts with fried onion and garlic as described, flavouring with thyme, then putting into a loaf tin or shallow casserole, and baking. This is good with cabbage or Brussels sprouts.

With their slight sweetness, cooked chestnuts can be made into some delicious puddings. Try puréeing them with apple juice concentrate and then folding in some thick yogurt or whipped cream, to make a luxurious fool. Or, for carob and chestnut truffles, mix 225 g/8 oz cooked mashed chestnuts with 1 tablespoon carob powder, a dash of vanilla essence and some apple juice concentrate, then roll small pieces of the mixture in carob powder.

PEANUT *Arachis hypogaea*

Neutral, nutrient

Peanuts contain many minerals and vitamins and are a good source of both nourishment and energy, useful during periods of extra physical work. Their B vitamin and phosphorus content makes peanuts a good strengthener and harmoniser of the nervous system, and some authors believe that they can calm without sedating.

Eaten with dates or figs, peanuts – like almonds – can create more moisture in the respiratory system, and are therefore useful for DRY COUGHS.

Note: Excessive consumption of peanuts can cause lethargy and contribute towards OBESITY. Whole peanuts should not be given to children under the age of about 5 or 6 because of the danger of choking. Smooth peanut butter is, however, quite safe and an excellent food for them.

Preparing and Using: Roasted peanuts are available almost everywhere; the disadvantage is that they are usually prepared with a large amount of added salt. Skinned peanuts are available from some supermarkets and also healthfood shops, where you can also buy peanut butter prepared without added salt, sugar or emulsifiers. The oil and solids usually separate when you store this type of peanut butter. Simply stir the mixture to re-incorporate the oil; or, for a lower-fat spread, pour off the oil and use it for cooking.

SAVOURY PEANUT SAUCE

This is a nourishing, protein-rich sauce. Pour it over steamed vegetables, including some potatoes, to make a complete meal. Serves 4.

> *6 tablespoons smooth or crunchy peanut butter*
> *lemon juice (optional)*
> *sea salt*

Put the peanut butter in a saucepan over a gentle heat and gradually mix in 300 ml/10 fl oz water. Simmer for a few minutes, stirring, until smooth and creamy. Add a dash of lemon juice, to taste if necessary, and a little salt.

PEANUT LOAF

This vegetarian savoury dish is rich in protein and makes an excellent replacement for meat or fish. Serve it with a MISO SAUCE (page 146) and steamed vegetables. Serves 4.

> *dried wholewheat breadcrumbs, to coat tin*
> *175 g/6 oz raw skinned peanuts*
> *2 tablespoons olive oil*
> *2 tablespoons peanut butter*
> *1 small onion, peeled and grated*
> *a small bunch of parsley*
> *175 g/6 oz cooked brown rice*
> *2 tablespoons shoyu or tamari*
> *sea salt*

Set the oven to 200°C/400°F/Gas Mark 6. Line a 450 g/1 lb loaf tin with greaseproof paper to cover the base and the narrow sides; grease well and sprinkle with the dried breadcrumbs. Fry the nuts in the oil for a few minutes until browned, stirring all the time. Mix well with the rest of the ingredients – this can be done in a food processor, chopping the nuts, onion and parsley at the same time. Add the rice, shoyu or tamari and seasoning. Mix thoroughly and spoon into the tin, pressing down well. Bake for 30 minutes, until firm and lightly browned.

PEANUT BURGERS

The above mixture also makes good burgers. Just form into burger shapes, coat in dried wholewheat breadcrumbs and shallow-fry in a little olive oil, or place on an oiled baking sheet and bake at 200°C/400°F/Gas Mark 6 for about 40 minutes until browned and crisp on both sides, turning the burgers after about 30 minutes.

PUMPKIN SEED *Cucurbita maxima*

Warming

Like other seeds and nuts, pumpkin seeds are rich in vitamins and minerals, particularly zinc, which makes them particularly valuable for GENITO-URINARY INFLAMMATIONS, including PROSTATE troubles. Anyone with these problems would find it helpful to eat a handful of de-husked pumpkin seeds each day; and some practitioners recommend that men should eat 10–12 pumpkin seeds each day as a precaution against them.

Pumpkin seeds are also renowned amongst herbalists for their ability to expel most worms from the intestine. During the day of treatment, no food should be eaten, except for a little CLEAR VEGETABLE BROTH (page 86) if desired. Take 40 g/1½ oz pumpkin seeds (preferably fresh), and 2 cloves garlic. Grind these to a pulp and divide the mixture into 3 portions. Take 1 dose for breakfast, 1 for lunch and 1 in the evening. Then take a herbal laxative mixture, which you can buy at a healthfood shop, before going to bed. Repeat this treatment after 5 days. Children aged 2–5 should have a third of the dose; those aged 6–12 should have half.

Preparing and Using: Pumpkin seeds can be bought plain, or salted and roasted. Whole, they can be eaten as a snack, added to fruit or vegetable salads, mueslis or crumble toppings.

To make a tasty pâté, grind or pulverise 50 g/2 oz pumpkin seeds, then mix with 2 teaspoons shoyu soy sauce and 2–3 teaspoons water, or a little more, to a thick, soft consistency. Crushed garlic or chopped spring onion can be added. This is good in sandwiches or on toast, or as a filling for small tomatoes with the seeds scooped out.

SAVOURY SEEDS

For a pleasant savoury snack, take equal quantities of pumpkin seeds, sunflower seeds and sesame seeds: say 1 tablespoon of each. Sprinkle with enough shoyu soy sauce to coat, mixing them so that the seeds are covered all over with shoyu. Spread them on a baking sheet and bake at 150°C/300°F/Gas Mark 2 for 15–20 minutes, or until dry and crisp.

SESAME SEED *Sesame indicum*

Neutral, tonic

Sesame seeds have numerous healing qualities and have been extensively used in the healing traditions of both China and India. They provide many minerals, particularly calcium, of which they are one of the best vegetable sources. As a result, sesame seeds strengthen the bones, nails and hair, slowing down the greying process; they are also reputed to strengthen the sight. They increase general vitality, improve the quality of the blood, and at the same time soothe the nervous system.

Eating sesame seeds strengthens WEAK YIN OF THE KIDNEYS and calms an OVERHEATED LIVER. They are excellent for CYSTITIS and other GENITO-URINARY INFLAMMATIONS and infections, especially when made into GOMASIO (see below).

Preparing and Using: Whole sesame seeds are widely available in healthfood shops, Middle Eastern shops and supermarkets. Sesame seed paste, or tahini, is available from healthfood shops and Middle Eastern shops. The pale type made by Cypressa has the most delicate flavour and is useful for making FAVOURITE HUMMUS (page 141). It can be spread on bread like peanut butter or mixed with water to make a nutritious milk.

Try powdering 50 g/2 oz sesame seeds, then mixing in 1 teaspoon honey, kneading the mixture and forming into small balls to make delicious halva sweets.

GOMASIO

One of the nicest ways of using sesame seeds is 10–15 parts roasted and ground with 1 part salt, to make gomasio. Makes 4–5 tablespoons.

> 10–15 *teaspoons sesame seeds*
> 1 *teaspoon sea salt*

Put the sesame seeds in a frying pan with the sea salt and dry roast over a moderate heat for a few minutes, stirring all the time, until the sesame seeds turn a slightly deeper brown and smell toasted. Powder the mixture with a pestle and mortar, or in an electric coffee grinder. This is delicious sprinkled over steamed vegetables, salads or baked potatoes, or even just on bread.

SUNFLOWER SEED *Heliantus annuus*

Warming, nourishing

Sunflower seeds are helpful for debilitated and cold lungs with a tendency to COLDS AND FLU, particularly during the winter. Their richness in nutrients, particularly B vitamins, makes them useful for a weak and stressed nervous system, and they increase sexual vigour both in men and women. Because of its high polyunsaturated fat content, sunflower seed oil is recommended for lowering cholesterol and reducing ATHERO-SCLEROSIS. It is also one of the best base oils, very good for massaging dry skins. For this purpose, and when the oil is to be used unheated, it is best to buy an organic, cold-pressed oil from a healthfood shop.

Preparing and Using: Sunflower seeds are widely available and, with their delicate flavour, can be used in many ways. They make an excellent milk (see below); can be added to cooked rice and salads; sprinkled over cooked vegetables; or made into a savoury nibble (see SAVOURY SEEDS, page 171).

SUNFLOWER MILK

This is a very pleasant white milk which is particularly good over breakfast cereals. Makes 750 ml/1¼ pints.

> *50 g/2 oz sunflower seeds*
> *honey (optional)*

Put the sunflower seeds in a food processor or liquidiser with 200 ml/7 fl oz water and whizz to a thick purée, then add another 400 ml/14 fl oz water and whizz again. Sweeten with a dash of honey if you like, and chill until needed.

WALNUT *Juglans regia*

Neutral

Most people are familiar with walnuts, but few realise the full medicinal value of the walnut tree, which includes the bark, leaves, oil and husks as well as the nuts themselves.

Like almonds, walnuts contain an abundance of vitamins and minerals. Eaten in moderation – say 10 a day – they can ease an OVERHEATED DIGESTION. Tea made from walnut leaves is tonic, astringent and diuretic, good for DIARRHOEA and for weak bowels; also, because of its ability to remove excess fluid, for OBESITY. The warm tea, used as a gargle, can help to tone up and soothe a SORE THROAT.

A similar tea, made from 2 teaspoons walnut leaves to 600 ml/1 pint water, can be used as a douche for VAGINAL DISCHARGES, using half the mixture in the morning and half in the evening. This treatment can be continued three times a week for a fortnight. This tea also makes a good enema for HAEMORRHOIDS (PILES); hold the water for as long as comfortable before discharging it. In addition the walnut leaf infusion makes an excellent final rinse when you're washing your hair, strengthening it and helping to slow down the greying process.

Powdered bark of the walnut tree can also be made into a tea as described; it is laxative and blood-cleansing. A tea made from the unripe husks of walnuts has blood-cleansing properties; it is antiseptic and can help expel worms from the intestines. And if the husks, leaves and shells of walnuts are left to infuse in a bucket of water for a few hours, the liquid can be drained off and used to spray the garden and keep slugs at bay.

Walnut oil is good for DRY, SCALY SKIN and, used as a massage oil, can stimulate and tonify a debilitated body.

Preparing and Using: Virtually all supermarkets sell walnut kernels, and walnuts in the shell during the winter months, and some sell walnut oil; otherwise this can be bought at delicatessens. Walnut leaves and bark can be obtained from herbalists.

To make tea from walnut leaves or bark, infuse 1 teaspoon crushed leaves or powdered bark in boiled water for 5–10 minutes. To make tea with the unripe husks, infuse 1 crushed husk in a cupful of boiled water for 5 minutes.

The nuts themselves, like other nuts and seeds, make good additions to salads, mueslis, cakes and biscuits. They can be made into milks and

174

creams and used to thicken sauces. And they are particularly tasty mixed with cooked brown rice and other grains, for added interest and nourishment, or made into a tasty stuffing for vegetables (see below).

WALNUT STUFFING FOR VEGETABLES

This is delicious on top of flat mushrooms, or as a filling for courgettes, marrows, aubergines or tomatoes. Makes enough to stuff 2 medium-sized courgettes.

> 1 *tablespoon olive oil*
> 1 *onion, peeled and chopped*
> 1 *garlic clove, peeled and crushed*
> 50 *g/2 oz walnuts*
> 1 *tomato, skinned, deseeded and chopped*
> *sea salt and freshly ground black pepper*

Heat the oil in a pan and sauté the onion and garlic for 10 minutes, until the onion is soft. If the vegetable you are stuffing has had some edible part removed to make room for the stuffing – courgettes, aubergines, or tomatoes, for instance – chop this roughly and add to the onion and garlic after 5 minutes, then cover and continue to cook for the remaining 5 minutes. Either chop the walnuts finely by hand and mix everything together; or put the onions and garlic in a food processor with the walnuts and the rest of the ingredients and whizz to a chunky purée. Season to taste with salt and pepper.

Fruit

As well as being a good source of vitamins and minerals, beautiful to look at, refreshing and tempting to the palate, fruit has many valuable healing properties. It's one of the pleasantest forms of 'medicine' available.

BUYING, STORING AND USING

Organically grown fruit is best when you can get it. If not, the skins should be well-scrubbed if they are going to be eaten, to remove all traces of sprays and waxes. Most fruit benefits from being kept in a cool place; soft fruits like grapes and strawberries keep best in the fridge.

Serve a single type of fruit or a mixture in a fruit salad; apple, orange or pineapple juice makes a good liquid for this instead of sugar syrup. Or try adding a little honey and water, or some apple juice concentrate; these are both delicious. For a sweeter mixture, include some dried fruits, especially dates and raisins.

Fruit is beneficial cooked as well as raw; in fact, for some conditions, it may be more appropriate served in this way. Again, honey, apple juice concentrate, a dash of Barbados sugar, or dried fruit can be used to sweeten the mixture. Sweet spices like ginger and cinnamon are also good in stewed or baked fruit dishes.

APPLE *Malus communis*

Cooling, cleansing

From earliest times, this lovely fruit has been praised by all schools of natural medicine. It cools and freshens the digestive system and blood, and is therefore useful for INDIGESTION with burning acidity, and for a variety of SKIN INFLAMMATIONS. Apples have the ability to harmonise the digestive system, helping both DIARRHOEA and CONSTIPATION. For diarrhoea, they are best eaten raw and grated; for constipation, cooked.

Apples were reputed to rest and strengthen the heart. According to Dr Binet, the French doctor and researcher, the pectin content of apples makes them useful for lowering cholesterol in the blood.

Apples soothe the kidneys and urinary system; they are mildly diuretic, helping the body to get rid of excess fluid and toxins. They are useful for OBESITY and, in particular, soothe the joints of sedentary people with a tendency to over-eating and/or to RHEUMATISM. Apples are one of the fruits that can be eaten by those who suffer from DIABETES.

Preparing and Using: Apples, like all fruits and vegetables, are most health-giving when organically grown and eaten with the skin still on. If you cannot get organically grown apples, scrub them well with hot water, to remove as much of the chemical residue as possible.

When buying apple juice, make sure it is pure, without added sugar. Apple juice concentrate (available at healthfood shops) is a good way of making up your own apple juice, as well as being an excellent natural sweetener.

For many cooking purposes, dessert apples are good because their natural sweetness means that no extra sugar is needed.

APPLE JELLY WITH MINT OR SAGE

This jelly is a delicious way of enjoying the healing properties of mint or sage, as well as those of apples. It's good with savoury pulse dishes, as well as with meats such as lamb; with cheese, or just on wholewheat bread. You can also make a rose petal version. For this, add 1 tablespoon dried rose petals, soaked and simmered until tender, or 3 tablespoons fresh scented rose petals (white inner part removed), simmered for a few minutes until tender. Add the rose petals with the apple juice concentrate, along with 1 tablespoon triple-distilled rose water instead of the cider vinegar. Makes about 175 g/6 oz.

> *450 g/1 lb cooking apples*
> *about 150 ml/5 fl oz apple juice concentrate*
> *juice of 1 lemon*
> *1 tablespoon cider vinegar*
> *2 tablespoons finely chopped fresh mint or sage*

Wash and quarter the apples, without peeling or coring. Put them in a saucepan with 300 ml/10 fl oz water. Simmer gently, with a lid on the pan, for about 20 minutes, or until the apples are very tender and mushy. Strain through a sieve, pushing through as much of the apple pulp as you can; make the amount up to 150 ml/5 fl oz with water if necessary and put this in a saucepan with the same quantity of apple juice concentrate, the lemon juice and cider vinegar. Boil for 10–15 minutes, or until the mixture looks thick and half a teaspoonful sets when chilled in the freezer for a few minutes. Add the chopped mint or sage, simmer for a few minutes longer, then remove from the heat and pour into a clear jar. Keep in the fridge.

SPICED BAKED APPLES WITH ALMONDS AND RAISINS

Cooking apples are excellent for baking and sweetness can be added with the filling. Preheat the oven to 200°C/400°F/Gas Mark 6. Score the apples round the middle, to stop them bursting, then scoop out the core. Fill the cavity with mixed raisins (lexia are wonderful when you can get them) and flaked or chopped almonds. Stick 3–4 cloves into each apple, then bake until soft (30–60 minutes, depending on the size of the apples). Serve with a little cream, nut cream or thick yogurt if you wish.

177

APRICOT *Prunus armeniaca*

Neutral, nourishing

Rich in vitamins and minerals, particularly in their dried form, apricots are an excellent fruit to nourish and improve the blood, recommended for ANAEMIA. They are also a good muscle tonic, their potassium and magnesium content giving strength and elasticity. In addition apricots – like apples – are helpful for dry CHEST INFLAMMATIONS.

Preparing and Using: Fresh apricots are available in season; dried apricots are easy to get all year round, but look for those which have been preserved without sulphur dioxide. They will look browner and less appetising, but taste delicious. The little Hunza apricots, which smell of brown sugar and taste wonderfully sweet, are the best of all. You can get these at healthfood shops. They are good just soaked for a few hours, then simmered gently until they are very tender and the water has reduced to a shiny syrup. Serve them as they are, with thick yogurt, cream or nut cream, or use them in the recipes below.

TOFU APRICOT FOOL

> 225–250 g/8–9 oz dried apricots
> 1 × 275 g/10 oz packet of silken tofu
> honey or apple juice concentrate

Soak and cook the dried apricots as described above. Then whizz them in a food processor or liquidiser with the tofu and a little honey or apple juice concentrate, to make a delicious creamy pudding.

HUNZA APRICOTS WITH ROSEWATER AND ALMONDS

This nourishing dish is good for the skin, for ANAEMIA and weakness, and for the chest. Serves 4.

> 450 g/1 lb Hunza apricots
> 1 tablespoon honey or apple juice concentrate
> 1–2 tablespoons rosewater
> 25 g/1 oz flaked almonds

Soak the apricots for several hours in cold water to cover. Then put them

178

in a pan with the honey or apple juice concentrate and enough soaking water to cover generously. (Top up with extra water if necessary.) Bring to the boil, and simmer gently for 30–40 minutes, or until the apricots are very tender and the water has reduced to a little syrup. If there is a great deal of water, remove the apricots to a dish, then boil the water until it has reduced to a syrup and pour this over the apricots. Serve warm or cold, sprinkled with the rosewater and almonds.

AVOCADO PEAR *Persea gratissima*

Neutral

Avocado pears are a very wholesome and nourishing food. They are rich in vitamins including carotene, vitamin E, the B vitamins (including folic acid) and vitamin C, as well as minerals such as potassium and iron. They soothe and strengthen the nervous system and are valuable during periods of overwork, both physical and mental. Their nourishing quality makes avocado pears helpful in times of convalescence and rapid growth. Dr Valnet writes that they can soothe the bladder in cases of CYSTITIS.

Preparing and Using: Make sure that the avocado pear is ripe; it should give to gentle pressure when cradled in your hand. Hard avocado pears ripen quickly if kept at room temperature for a few days. Once ready to eat, keep them in the salad compartment of the fridge to prevent them from getting over-ripe.

Avocado pear can be eaten halved and sprinkled with lemon juice, olive oil and seasoning; or it can be sliced into a vegetable or fruit salad, to add creamy texture and richness. You may enjoy sliced avocado on bread, toast or crispbread, as a nourishing snack. It is also good as a sandwich filling, mixed with salad ingredients such as lettuce, grated carrot, tomato, cucumber, perhaps a few sprouted mung beans (see page 138) and chopped fresh herbs; or whizzed into a creamy dip (see below).

CREAMY AVOCADO DIP

There are many versions of this dip, which also makes an excellent non-dairy mayonnaise-type dressing for salad. Serves 4.

1 *ripe avocado, halved and stoned*
1 *garlic clove, peeled*
1 *green chilli, deseeded*
½ *green pepper, deseeded*
a few sprigs of fresh coriander, mint or basil
1 *tomato, skinned*
juice of ½–1 *lemon or lime*
sea salt and freshly ground black pepper

Scoop out the avocado flesh and mash it, or whizz it in a food processor, with some or all of the above ingredients. Season to taste with salt and pepper, and serve with crudités or pitta bread if you wish.

AVOCADO, BANANA, CAROB AND HONEY SPREAD

This rich, creamy spread makes an excellent snack during times of overwork, NERVOUS TENSION or strenuous sporting activity. It is particularly good spread on crisp OATCAKES (see page 160) as oats are also soothing to the nervous system. This mixture is also delicious served as a pudding; spoon the mixture into a small ramekin or other suitable container and chill well – or even freeze lightly – before serving. Again, it's good accompanied by an oaty biscuit. Serves 1.

½ *small ripe banana*
¼ *large ripe avocado*
2 *teaspoons carob powder*
1–2 *teaspoons honey*
a few drops of real vanilla essence (optional)

Peel the banana and the avocado, then mash them together with the carob powder, honey, and vanilla essence if using, until you get a creamy consistency.

BANANA *Musa spp.*

Cooling, nourishing

Banana, with its high starch and carbohydrate content and its many nutrients, is a good food for times when you're burning up a great deal of energy. In addition, bananas have a mild calming effect on the nervous system, so they are useful when there is STRESS due to overwork, either physical or mental. Dried bananas are considered helpful in relieving CONSTIPATION.

Note: Bananas should not be eaten by people with DIABETES or by those with a cold and sluggish metabolism and a tendency to OBESITY and lethargy.

Preparing and Using: Bananas taste best when the skins are speckled with brown; they can be kept at room temperature for several days to reach this stage. They make a wonderfully convenient snack; are good baked whole for about 20 minutes; or sliced and served with brown sugar, honey or maple syrup and cream or yogurt; or added to fruit salads. Sliced bananas also make a good accompaniment to some curries and spiced rice dishes.

For a delicious treat, rather like a healthy choc-ice, try dipping chunks of banana first in clear honey, then in carob powder and finally in chopped nuts. Put them in the freezer until firm.

BANANA WITH CAROB SAUCE

This is a delicious combination – a quick-to-make, indulgent yet healthy pudding. The sauce can be used over other fruits, yogurt or ice-cream. Serves 1.

> 1 tablespoon carob powder
> 2 tablespoons maple syrup or apple juice concentrate
> 10 g / ¼ oz butter
> ½ teaspoon real vanilla essence
> 1 banana
> a few chopped nuts (optional)

Put the carob in a small saucepan with the maple syrup or apple juice concentrate, the butter and vanilla essence, and mix well. Heat gently, stirring, until smooth. Peel and slice the banana and put into a serving bowl. Pour the sauce over the top, sprinkle with the chopped nuts if using, and serve.

BILBERRY *Vaccinium myrtillus*

Cool, moist and cleansing

These tiny purple berries, also known as blueberries, are charged with energy and healing qualities. They are perhaps valued most highly by practitioners of natural medicine for their ability to strengthen the eyes and improve the quality of vision. They cool, cleanse and strengthen the liver, kidneys and blood (getting rid of uric acid and cholesterol deposits) and the system in general. These actions make bilberries valuable, especially for sedentary people who tend to accumulate toxins and could have painful, INFLAMED JOINTS and irritated DRY SKIN. They are also helpful for HEART DISEASE and CIRCULATORY PROBLEMS.

Bilberries are very good for what the Chinese call TOO LITTLE YIN and are recommended for FEVERS when there is a great deal of heat, redness and thirst. They moisten and cleanse the intestines and in laboratory tests in France have been shown to inhibit many bacteria which can cause putrefaction and inflammation in the digestive tract. Bilberries also relieve CONSTIPATION, especially when this is associated with dry stools and HAEMORRHOIDS (PILES).

They are helpful for MOUTH ULCERS. For these you can either take them internally or use the juice as a mouth wash; or you can chew the berries very slowly, keeping them in your mouth for as long as possible.

Some healthfood shops sell bilberry juice, or might be persuaded to order it for you. Drink half a glass diluted to taste with water, sipping it throughout the day. The dry berries are also sometimes available and can be made into a tea.

The leaves are used by some medical herbalists as a tea to treat pancreatic disturbances and DIABETES, and to strengthen the circulation and the capillaries. They are mildly diuretic and a cleanser of the urinary system, and also help to relieve DIARRHOEA.

Preparing and Using: Bilberries are good eaten raw, or stewed over a gentle heat with some clear honey or apple juice concentrate: 2–3 tablespoons honey, or 4 tablespoons apple juice concentrate, to 450 g/ 1 lb bilberries. They are excellent served with thick yogurt; or you could try sieving them and folding them into some yogurt to make a fool.

BLACKCURRANT *Ribes nigrum*

Cooling

These berries have similar properties to those of bilberries, though perhaps in a slightly milder form. The leaves are sometimes used as a tea, for their cool, dry action on red, painful and swollen joints due to RHEUMATISM. They are mildly diuretic.

Preparing and Using: Blackcurrants need topping and tailing, unless they are going to be sieved. Cook them as described for bilberries. They make one of the best jams or jellies; you can buy no-added sugar blackcurrant jam, or make your own. Simply stew blackcurrants in the minimum of water until tender, then add the same volume of apple juice concentrate and the juice of a lemon. Boil until a teaspoon of the mixture sets when chilled in the freezer for a few minutes. Bottle and keep in the fridge.

CHERRY *Cerasus vulgaris*

Neutral, cleansing

For centuries cherries have been renowned in the West as one of the best fruits and vegetables for cleansing of the body. They remove toxins and fluids, clean the kidneys and give a rosy complexion. Their cleansing properties make them valuable in the treatment of RHEUMATISM and GOUT, and their mild laxative action is useful for CONSTIPATION. They soothe the nervous system, refreshing the mind and relieving STRESS. In ancient times, cherries were believed, both in the East and West, to rejuvenate the body.

The stalks of cherries are more warming than the fruits. When made into a tea they have a very good diuretic action which is helpful for CYSTITIS and for GENITO-URINARY INFECTIONS and discharges. They also have a mildly astringent effect on the intestines, relieving DIARRHOEA.

Preparing and Using: Cherries are delectable as they are, made into a compote, or added to a fruit salad. For a delicious soup, stone some black cherries and put them in a saucepan. Cover with water or red wine and add a piece of broken cinnamon stick. Simmer until the cherries are tender. Then liquidise some of the mixture and add it to the rest, to thicken the soup. Sweeten with honey or apple juice concentrate. Chill, then serve in chilled bowls with a swirl of soured cream and a sprinkling of powdered cinnamon on each portion.

BLACK CHERRY AND CINNAMON COMPOTE

Serves 4.

> 750 g/1½ lb black cherries, halved and stoned
> a piece of cinnamon stick
> juice and grated rind of ½ well-scrubbed unwaxed orange
> 4 tablespoons apple juice concentrate

183

Put all the ingredients in a heavy-based saucepan and cook gently for about 5 minutes, until the cherries are soft and the liquid syrupy. Serve hot or cold, with thick yogurt if you wish.

DATE *Phoenix dactylifera*

Neutral, nutrient

These deliciously sweet fruits are rich in minerals such as magnesium, calcium and copper which strengthen the nervous system whilst at the same time giving extra energy and endurance. Dates lubricate the lungs and are useful for DRY COUGHS and SORE THROATS.

Note: Dates should not be eaten by those suffering from DIABETES, HYPOGLYCAEMIA or OBESITY.

Preparing and Using: Fresh dates are the most delicious, when you can get them. They make a wonderful natural treat, eaten just as they are, or with the stone removed and replaced with a nut or piece of marzipan. Or they can be sliced and added to fruit salads and compotes. Dried dates are almost as good and can be used as a tasty sugar replacement in cakes. Choose dates which have not had any extra sugar added.

DATE SLICES

Served hot or warm, perhaps with some thick Greek yogurt or single cream, these make a lovely pudding. Cold, they're a sweet and delicious cake. They're good for the nervous system, especially when served with the ALMOND CREAM on page 167. Makes 14.

> *150 g/5 oz butter or margarine*
> *175 g/6 oz rolled oats*
> *100 g/4 oz plain wholewheat flour*
> *225 g/8 oz stoned dates*
> *1 tablespoon lemon juice*
> *1 tablespoon honey*
> *a dash of real vanilla essence*

Set the oven to 180°C/350°F/Gas Mark 4. Grease an 18 cm/7 in square tin with a little of the butter or margarine. Put the oats and flour in a bowl and rub in the rest of the butter or margarine, then press half the mixture into the tin. Simmer the dates in 2 tablespoons water over a gentle heat for about 10 minutes, until soft. Remove from the heat and stir in the lemon juice, honey and vanilla essence. Spread this over the oat mixture in the tin, then cover with the rest of the oat mixture and press down firmly. Bake for about 25 minutes, until golden brown. Cut into bars while still warm, then leave to cool in the tin.

FIG *Ficus carica*

Cooling, nourishing, laxative

Raw figs are soothing and healing, both to the respiratory system, where they can help DRY COUGHS and inflamed conditions, and to the digestive system, for hot and inflamed conditions such as ULCERS, acidity and HEARTBURN. They have a marked action on the intestines, being very therapeutic for ailments such as DIVERTICULITIS, CONSTIPATION and HAEMOR-RHOIDS (PILES). Whilst being soothing to eat and easy to digest, figs are also a rich source of vitamins and minerals, and are therefore an excellent food for convalescents, children and old people.

Dried figs contain more vitamins and minerals – such as carotene, folic acid, B vitamins, potassium and calcium – than fresh figs. They are also a good source of natural sugars, and thus useful during physical activity.

Note: Dried figs are not advised for those with DIABETES or for people with a SLOW DIGESTION.

Preparing and Using: Fresh figs, when available, are incomparable. They should be soft to the touch but not wet-looking or bruised. Slice and serve them on their own, or mix them with other fruits in compotes and fruit salads. They are excellent with a soft white cheese, such as ricotta; try slicing the figs down from the top three times, then pulling the sections back to resemble petals and filling the centre of the 'flower' with a little cream cheese.

Dried figs are a wonderful natural sweetener; just 1–2 stewed with tart fruits such as apples will not only add a delicious flavour but also mean that other sweeteners can be cut to the minimum or done away with altogether. They can be used or eaten as they are, or, particularly if being added to a fruit compote, soaked for a few hours before use.

FIGS WITH PRUNES, PEARS AND APPLES

This dish is particularly good for anyone suffering from CONSTIPATION, but it is delicious to eat any time. Serves 2.

6 dried figs
6 prunes
1–2 eating apples
1 large pear (preferably Conference)
3 cloves (optional)
a small piece of cinnamon stick (optional)
2 teaspoons apple juice concentrate or honey (optional)

Cover the figs and prunes with water and soak for a few hours, or overnight. Wash the apples and pear, and cut, unpeeled, into thick slices, discarding the cores. Put the apple and pear slices in a saucepan with the figs, prunes, cloves and cinnamon if using, and 300 ml/10 fl oz water. Bring to the boil and boil for 2–3 minutes. Then simmer over a low heat, without a lid on the pan, for 40–50 minutes, or until the fruits are very tender and most of the water has evaporated, leaving a glossy syrup. Remove the cloves and cinnamon stick if used. Add the honey or apple juice concentrate if necessary. Serve hot, warm or cold, perhaps with thick yogurt.

GRAPE *Vitis vinifera*

Neutral to cooling, cleansing, nourishing

Some Chinese authors describe grapes as having a warming energy, but what they are really describing is the wine, rather than the fruit. Throughout the Mediterranean, grapes have always been highly regarded, not only for their tonic quality and usefulness during periods of STRESS and overwork, but also for their cleansing action. With their high mineral and vitamin content and natural sugars, grapes – especially the red or purple varieties – are indeed a good tonic and blood-builder. They cleanse the blood, eliminate OEDEMA (FLUID RETENTION), clean a congested body, remove CONSTIPATION and cool an OVERHEATED LIVER. Grapes are also reputed to help slightly with HYPERTENSION (HIGH BLOOD PRESSURE).

Grapes are even more energising in their dried form, as raisins. These are fortifying at times of heavy physical work and during sport. They also soothe inflamed and irritated lungs, and DRY COUGHS.

186

Note: Like other dried fruits, raisins are not advised for those suffering from DIABETES and other sugar metabolism problems.

Preparing and Using: The many different varieties of this fruit ensure a year-round supply. Wash grapes thoroughly to remove dust and spray residues; halve them and remove the seeds before adding to fruit mixtures or vegetable salads. Perhaps the most delicious raisins are lexia, with muscatels also ranking highly. Less luscious varieties are good when 'plumped' by covering them with boiling water and leaving them to stand for half an hour before draining.

FRUIT CAKE WITHOUT ADDED SUGAR

This recipe is a slightly modified version of the one given in *Rose Elliot's Complete Vegetarian Cookbook*. It contains no added sugar, fat or eggs. Makes 1 × 1 kg/2 lb loaf.

> *225 g/8 oz cooking dates (not sugar-rolled)*
> *175 g/6 oz raisins*
> *100 g/4 oz sultanas*
> *100 g/4 oz currants*
> *50 g/2 oz candied mixed peel, chopped*
> *175 g/6 oz plain 100% wholewheat flour*
> *1 tablespoon carob powder (optional)*
> *3 teaspoons baking powder*
> *1 teaspoon mixed spice*
> *grated rind of 1 orange or lemon*
> *25 g/1 oz ground almonds*
> *a few flaked almonds*

Set the oven to 160°C/325°F/Gas Mark 3. Grease a 1 kg/2 lb loaf tin and line with greased greaseproof or non-stick paper. Put the dates in a saucepan with 300 ml/10 fl oz water and heat gently until they are soft. Remove from the heat and mash to a purée. Put the date purée in a bowl with the raisins, sultanas, currants, mixed peel, flour, carob powder if using, baking powder, spice, grated rind, ground almonds and 4 table-spoons water. Mix well, then spoon into the tin and level the top. Sprinkle with the flaked almonds and bake for about 1½ hours, or until a skewer inserted into the centre comes out clean. Allow to cool a little in the tin, then turn the cake out and finish cooling on a wire rack.

187

GRAPEFRUIT *Citrus decumana*

Cooling, cleansing, beneficial to the liver

Grapefruit has a strongly cleansing and regenerating action on a congested and OVERHEATED LIVER. It also cleanses the urinary system and is diuretic (qualities which are similar to those of pineapple). Like other citrus fruits such as oranges, lemons, limes and tangerines, grapefruit helps the digestive system to break down fats; it is therefore good to eat after a rich meal, especially one high in animal fat. These two qualities – the ability to get rid of excess fluid and to break down fat – make grapefruit especially valuable for WEIGHT LOSS. In addition, grapefruit helps to clear putrefaction from the intestines and to get rid of CONSTIPATION.

Grapefruit purifies and cools the blood and joints, improving SKIN INFLAMMATIONS and RHEUMATISM. It helps to eliminate mucus from the respiratory system and from the body generally; it cools FEVERS and COLDS with a predominance of heat and inflammation.

BROKEN CAPILLARIES are helped and healed by grapefruit which is also recommended for CIRCULATORY PROBLEMS, ATHEROSCLEROSIS and HYPERTENSION (HIGH BLOOD PRESSURE).

Preparing and Using: Always weigh grapefruits in your hands before buying them; the heavier they feel, the better.

To use them in fruit and salad mixtures, try cutting the grapefruit segments away from the skin and the pith, cutting the peel off at the top and going round and round, as you do when removing the skin of an apple in a single piece. Then cut each segment away from the inner transparent skin. The juicy pieces of grapefruit are delicious mixed with orange sections prepared in the same way, and some chopped mint; with slices of avocado pear, or with watercress and a sprinkling of sesame seeds. A mixture of ordinary grapefruit and pink grapefruit works well.

To cleanse the liver and help to cure CONSTIPATION, put thick pieces of the peel (perhaps saved from the above) and a little of the pulp in a saucepan, cover with water and boil for a few minutes. Strain, and drink the juice, with a dash of lemon juice and a little honey, sugar or apple juice concentrate added if you wish.

Eating 1–2 teaspoons no-added sugar marmalade made from grapefruit peel is also a good remedy for LIVER PROBLEMS. And essential oil of grapefruit, mixed with a base oil, has a similar action when massaged over the abdomen.

188

LEMON AND LIME *Citrus limon and Citrus aurantifolia*

Cooling, cleansing, tonic, antiseptic

Lemons are endowed with many healing qualities; and they are one of the natural medicines which the eminent French naturopath, Dr Valnet, values most. Nutritionally lemons are noted for their high vitamin C content; they increase resistance to infections and may strengthen the immune system. They also have antiseptic properties which were interestingly demonstrated in a study in which lemon juice was poured over shellfish: the lemon juice eliminated 92 per cent of their bacteria within 15 minutes.

For all these reasons lemons are invaluable for COLDS, FLU and BRONCHITIS; they cool FEVERS and help the respiratory system get rid of bacteria and mucus. The antiseptic properties of lemons act on the digestive system, eliminating putrefaction and harmful bacteria, helping the assimilation of nutrients and the elimination of toxins. The urinary system, too, benefits from the antiseptic action of lemons, which can help with problems such as CYSTITIS.

Lemons have a positive, healing action on the liver and the blood, cleansing and restoring a toxic and OVERHEATED LIVER which can create problems such as nausea, bitter taste in the mouth and HEADACHES; purifying the blood, eliminating cholesterol and keeping the blood more fluid. This benefits the circulatory system, and also the skin, which becomes clearer. Lemons help the system get rid of mucus and fats and are thus valuable for WEIGHT LOSS. In addition, lemons are useful for RHEUMATISM, especially when the joints are hot, swollen and painful; and they are considered to be a tonic for the nervous system.

Essential oil of lemon is highly antiseptic; studies by Morel and Rochaix have shown that its vapours can sterilise many highly potent bacteria, such as meningococcus and staphylococcus, within a few minutes.

Preparing and Using: Buy organic or unwaxed lemons if you want to use the skins, and scrub well. As with all citrus fruit, you should choose those which feel heavy in your hand.

For lemon tea, put 1 teaspoon grated rind in a cup, top up with freshly boiled water and leave to infuse for 5 minutes. Alternatively, you could boil a slice of lemon in water for 5 minutes, then strain into a cup.

A teaspoonful of fresh lemon juice added to a cupful of warm water makes an effective gargle for all infections of the mouth and throat.

For COLDS AND FLU, add the juice of ½ lemon or 1 whole lime to a cupful of boiling water and sweeten to taste with honey. Drink 3 of these cups a day.

Lemon juice is an indispensable ingredient in the kitchen, for both sweet and savoury dishes. It is good poured over cooked or raw vegetables, perhaps with some fruity olive oil; sprinkled over fruit salads, to help preserve the colour of delicate fruits, as well as to add flavour; brushed over the cut surfaces of artichokes, again, to prevent them from discolouring; served with FAVOURITE HUMMUS (page 141) or POLENTA (page 156); in herb teas; or to flavour fruit cakes.

MANDARIN, TANGERINE *Citrus nobilis, Citrus reticulata*

Neutral

Although milder, the main action of mandarins and tangerines is similar to that of oranges, benefiting the general defences of the body and of particular value for COLDS AND FLU. In addition, mandarins and tangerines are helpful for DIARRHOEA and loose stools, soothing irritated intestines; healing inflamed lungs and expectorating mucus; they are also mildly relaxing. The dry peel of tangerines, which is slightly warming, is used as a tea in Chinese medicine to alleviate STAGNATION OF ENERGY IN THE LIVER, to reduce diarrhoea and to expel mucus from the lungs.

Preparing and Using: Children's favourites, and ideal for popping into lunch boxes, these fruits also make excellent additions to fruit salads. Buy bright, firm mandarins and tangerines, and try combining them with sliced kiwi fruits and lychees for an interesting contrast of colours, flavours and textures.

MANGO *Mangifera indica*

Neutral, moist

A favourite fruit in India to sweeten the mouth and quench the thirst, mango helps an OVERHEATED DIGESTION and has a mildly soothing and calming action on the nervous system, thus also easing nervous INDIGESTION. Mango is especially good for thin, nervous people who are over-active and tend to feel hot. It calms their body, mind and emotions whilst at the same time giving them energy. Mango is also mildly diuretic and laxative.

190

Note: Those with DIABETES, excessive mucus in the system or a SLOW DIGESTION should take care not to eat too much mango.

Preparing and Using: Mango gives a little to the touch when ripe, and smells fragrant. To prepare it, stand the mango on a board with the stalk end uppermost. With a sharp, stainless steel knife, cut straight down the mango about 5 mm/¼ in to the side of the stalk. Repeat this procedure on the other side of the stalk, then cut the flesh away from the large stone. Remove the peel from the pieces of mango and slice the flesh.

A sweet ripe mango is delectable on its own with no embellishments. But if you like, you could slice 2–3 mangoes, then liquidise some of the flesh with some water to make a thin sauce, and add this to the sliced mangoes. You can also make a wonderfully sweet and filling drink by liquidising peeled mango with enough water, orange juice or apple juice to get a pouring consistency. This drink, frozen, then broken up into rough chunks and whizzed in a food processor makes a delicious sorbet.

FRUIT SALAD WITH MANGO SAUCE

Serves 4.

> 1 *medium-sized ripe mango*
> 225 *g/8 oz strawberries, hulled and halved*
> 2 *kiwi fruits, peeled and sliced*
> 225 *g/8 oz black grapes, halved and deseeded*
> 1 *pawpaw or piece of melon, sliced, with peel and seeds removed*
> *a few fresh mint leaves, to decorate*

Halve the mango, removing the skin and stone. Cut the flesh into chunks and liquidise to a smooth purée, adding a little water to get the consistency of single cream. Pour this sauce on to 4 plates, arrange the fruits on top, decorate with fresh mint leaves, and serve.

MELON *Cucumis melo*

Cooling, cleansing, anti-inflammatory

Melon, like pawpaw, is one of the most anti-inflammatory fruits. Very refreshing and soothing to all systems, it cools an OVERHEATED DIGESTION with symptoms such as DYSPEPSIA, GASTRITIS, ULCERS, ACIDITY, COLITIS and both dry CONSTIPATION and burning DIARRHOEA. Melon not only calms fire in the stomach but also an OVERHEATED LIVER; it soothes urinary problems

191

such as mild KIDNEY INFLAMMATIONS and CYSTITIS; and can ease inflamed joints due to RHEUMATISM. Melon can also be crushed and applied externally to heal inflamed and sore skin, and also to refresh and rejuvenate it.

Preparing and Using: When they are ripe, scented melons like ogen and charentais smell fragrant and the stem gives a little. Tough-skinned honeydew melons are less easy to judge; one way of ensuring that they are ripe is to keep them for several days at room temperature. A really sweet, ripe, juicy melon is delicious and needs no accompaniments; indeed, those who follow a food-combining diet maintain that melon is not easy to digest when mixed with any other foods.

A melon which is less than perfect can be cheered up with a sprinkling of powdered cinnamon or ginger. Or you could dice the flesh and marinate the chunks with clear honey or apple juice concentrate, some cinnamon stick, crushed cardomom pods, sprigs of rosemary, leaves of lemon verbena or mint.

ORANGE *Citrus aurantium*

Cooling, cleansing

The orange tree offers healing gifts in abundance: from its leaves and flowers; and from the flesh, juice and peel of its fruit. The fruit is rich in vitamin C and so, like lemons, is helpful for the prevention and treatment of COLDS AND FLU, especially when these are accompanied by a raised temperature, and a feeling of heat rather than chilliness. Like lemons and also grapefruits, oranges are useful in helping to expel hot and yellow mucus from the respiratory system and other parts of the body.

Oranges cool the digestion and are helpful for hot and acid stomachs. Again, like grapefruits and lemons, oranges cool and cleanse the blood, clearing cholesterol from the arteries; and they contribute towards a healthy skin. They are useful for BROKEN CAPILLARIES; for red and hot extremities; for HYPERTENSION (HIGH BLOOD PRESSURE), ATHEROSCLEROSIS and THROMBOSIS.

The peel of oranges works on the stomach, liver and intestines to relieve what the Chinese describe as stagnant energy, the symptoms of which are abdominal swelling and soreness, soreness over the liver area, hiccups, belching, flatulence and CONSTIPATION. A tea made with 1 teaspoon dried peel of bitter oranges is extremely helpful for these conditions. Alternatively, you could eat 1–2 teaspoons of a no-added sugar chunky marmalade with breakfast and after main meals.

A tea made from 1 teaspoon orange flowers works in a gentle, calming and soothing way on the nervous system. It is helpful for nervous HEADACHES and INDIGESTION; for TENSION, STRESS and INSOMNIA. Just being near fragrant orange blossom in the spring can be uplifting to the spirit, cheering and relaxing to the mind and body.

A highly aromatic and expensive essential oil called neroli is extracted from orange flowers. It is extremely soothing to the nervous system, either diluted in a base oil and used for massage, or added to the bath. You could also sprinkle a few drops on a cotton handkerchief or on your pillow.

Another essential oil is extracted from the leaves of the orange tree. This is called petit grain and, like neroli, works on the nervous system, but in a more stimulating tonic way. It is also less costly.

Note: Modern studies indicate that in certain people excessive consumption of oranges can disturb the liver.

Preparing and Using: Oranges of different types are available throughout the year – the navel oranges are perhaps the best. As with any citrus fruit, choose ones which feel heavy. Dried orange peel and flowers can be bought from herbalists; and the essential oils from the suppliers listed on page 281.

Oranges are delicious when freshly squeezed, or cut into skinless segments as described for grapefruit (page 188) and served as they are or mixed into fruit or fresh vegetable salads. The grated peel of well-scrubbed unwaxed oranges makes a useful flavouring for many dishes, both sweet and savoury – try it with cooked beetroot, carrot, pumpkin or sweet potato. Or make a salad of sliced orange, grated orange rind, watercress and onion rings. Sliced radishes and orange rings are another colourful and refreshing combination, as is celery or chicory, orange and chopped walnuts.

PAWPAW, PAPAYA *Carica papaya*

Neutral to cooling, emollient, anti-inflammatory

Pawpaw cools the body and reduces inflammation; it is valuable for soothing digestive ULCERS, GASTRITIS, burning DIARRHOEA, DIVERTICULITIS and so on. It cools an OVERHEATED LIVER with symptoms such as red eyes and face, 'bursting' HEADACHES and irritability. Pawpaw is useful during

FEVERS, when there is much sweating and heat. In fact pawpaw is probably one of the best cooling, softening and anti-inflammatory foods of all. Whenever there is redness, burning and dryness in the system, think first of pawpaw.

As a treatment for SKIN INFLAMMATIONS, apply a thin slice of pawpaw, with its peel, to the affected area for several hours. Injections of pawpaw extract have been found to be effective in helping INFLAMED DISCS.

Pawpaw also has a calming effect on sexual desire. (Some monasteries in the Far East give large portions of pawpaw to the monks and nuns as an anaphrodisiac.) So do not eat too much of it when you want all your loving ardour intact.

If a meat stew is cooked with a piece of pawpaw leaf added, the leaf will tenderise the meat.

Preparing and Using: As they ripen, pawpaws become tinged with yellow, fragrant, and yielding to the touch. Cut the pawpaw in half and scoop the shiny round black seeds away from the pink flesh. The flesh can be eaten from the cut halves with a teaspoon; or the pawpaw can be peeled and sliced. Pawpaw makes a colourful addition to fruit salad mixtures.

PAWPAW WITH SCENTED GERANIUM LEAVES

Serves 2–3.

> 2 *ripe pawpaws*
> 6–8 *large scented geranium leaves, plus 2–3 small ones to decorate*

Peel the pawpaws, scoop out the seeds, and slice the flesh. Line a shallow dish with 3–4 torn geranium leaves; put the slices of pawpaw on top, then cover with more leaves. Put a plate and a light weight on top and leave for 2 hours or so. Remove the leaves; divide the pawpaw between individual bowls and decorate each with a small fresh scented geranium leaf.

PEACH *Prunus persica*

Cooling, digestive, laxative

There has been some confusion about the properties of this fruit because some writers have thought that information given in ancient texts about peach kernels referred to the peaches themselves. Peach kernels are warming, whereas the fruit cools and moistens the body. Peaches

194

cleanse the system, purifying the blood and giving a clear skin. Crushed ripe peaches, applied to the face for a few minutes each day, can help to keep the skin cool, fresh and youthful.

Peaches are useful for CONSTIPATION with dry stools, burning INDIGESTION and inflamed, DRY SKIN. They also have a diuretic action and are therefore helpful for WEIGHT LOSS and OEDEMA (FLUID RETENTION). Peaches have a mild, soothing effect on the nervous system and heart and can also help to lower cholesterol and prevent or reduce ATHEROSCLEROSIS.

The flowers can be made into a tea which calms and promotes sound sleep. And dried peaches, available at healthfood shops, are a concentrated source of nourishment, rich in iron and other minerals.

Preparing and Using: Ripe peaches can be used with or without their skin. To remove the skin, put the peaches in a bowl and cover with boiling water. Leave for a couple of minutes, then see if the skin will come off; if not, leave for a bit longer. Slice the peaches and remove the stones. Peaches prepared like this can be marinated in sweet white wine for several hours or overnight, added to fruit salad mixtures, or included in salads. They are particularly good combined with soft white cheeses.

Try a fruit salad made from sliced fresh peaches, soaked and lightly cooked dried peaches, and flaked almonds. Ripe peaches can also be sliced and whizzed in a food processor with cream or yogurt to make fools and ice-creams.

PEAR *Pirus communis*

Cool

Pears can cool and calm a nervous, inflamed and acidic digestive system; they are useful in conditions such as GASTRITIS, ACIDITY, nervous DYSPEPSIA, COLITIS, IRRITABLE BOWEL SYNDROME and DIVERTICULITIS. As they are slightly diuretic and can also help to regulate the intestines, they are helpful both for DIARRHOEA and CONSTIPATION. Pears can help reduce inflammation in hot and swollen joints due to RHEUMATISM and they are also prescribed to soothe the COUGHS and spasms of an irritated respiratory system. Dried pears, which you can get at healthfood shops, are delicious.

Preparing and Using: It's a good idea to buy hard pears and let them ripen at room temperature, so that they are perfect when you eat them. Once ripe, they will keep for 1–2 days in the fridge.

Peel and core the pears, then slice; or peel under-ripe pears and poach gently in water and honey until very tender. Sliced pears are also good cooked in honey in a covered dish in the oven.

HONEYED PEARS WITH ANISEED

To calm COUGHS and moisten dry lungs. Serves 1.

> 1 *pear, cored and sliced*
> 1 *dried fig*
> 1 *date*
> ½ *teaspoon aniseed*
> 1 *teaspoon honey*

Put all the ingredients in a saucepan with enough water to cover. Bring to the boil and simmer for 45 minutes, until the fruits are very tender and the liquid has reduced to a shiny syrup.

PINEAPPLE *Ananas comosus*

Cool, moist, anti-inflammatory

Pineapple, like pawpaw, is one of the best anti-inflammatory agents in nature. It is both demulcent (soothing inflammations inside the body) and emollient (soothing them outside). It calms an OVERHEATED DIGESTION and is useful during FEVERS when there is much sweating and heat. Pineapple greatly helps inflammation in the female reproductive system, improving both DYSMENORRHOEA (PAINFUL MENSTRUATION) and MENORRHAGIA (EXCESSIVE MENSTRUATION). It cools the blood and clears the skin, keeping it fresh and youthful. For this purpose you can also use pineapple externally, washing your face with a slice of pineapple or its juice. Pineapple is also very good for weight loss.

Note: Because it is rather acidic, pineapple is not recommended for over-acidic digestions.

Preparing and Using: A ripe pineapple smells sweet and syrupy, and one of the inner leaves will pull out easily. When preparing pineapple, you should always cut out all the 'eyes'. A good, simple way of serving a medium-sized pineapple is to cut it into 4–6 slices from top to bottom, keeping the leaves attached to each slice for decoration. Cut away the central core if it is tough (this is not always necessary). Then cut the sections across into segments and loosen them by cutting between them and the skin, being careful to keep them still in place.

Small pineapples can be halved in a similar manner, then the flesh can be scooped out, chopped and mixed with other fruits such as strawberries or grapes before being replaced. Pineapple is good mixed with creamy ingredients such as avocado or cream cheese.

PINEAPPLE JELLY

This is cooling and soothing, good for inflamed digestive conditions. It is impossible to make jelly from fresh pineapple with gelatine (derived from hooves and bones) because of the action of the enzymes in the pineapple on the protein in the gelatine. But with a vegetable jelling agent there is no problem. Serves 6.

> 1 *small pineapple, peeled, cored and diced*
> 2 *teaspoons gelozone*
> 600 *ml/1 pint natural pineapple juice*

Divide the pineapple chunks between 6 dishes. Put the gelozone in a saucepan and mix to a paste with a little of the pineapple juice. Gradually stir in the rest of the juice, and heat gently until the mixture almost boils, stirring all the time. Cool slightly, then pour over the pineapple. The mixture will set quite quickly as it cools.

PLUM *Prunus domestica*

Neutral, laxative, digestive

Plums cleanse and regenerate the liver, especially when it is too hot. They also cool the stomach and intestines which are sometimes affected by an OVERHEATED LIVER. For this, both raw and cooked plums are the most important fruit to cool the digestion, and remove stagnant abdominal energy with symptoms of bloating, swelling and flatulence. Plums also cleanse and cool the blood, helping to keep the skin fresh and youthful. In addition Dr Valnet states that they soothe and strengthen the nervous system.

Dried plums, in the form of prunes, are a very good source of iron, as well as calcium, magnesium and phosphorus. Prunes can help CONSTIPA-TION, particularly if you boil them and then drink the water as well as eating the fruit. A good remedy for constipation is made by soaking 8 prunes overnight; then, next morning, add 8 fresh plums, 1 teaspoon fennel seeds, water to cover and some cinnamon to taste, and boil for 45 minutes. The mixture should be eaten over a period of 3 days.

The water in which prunes are cooked is effective as a diuretic, to ease OEDEMA (FLUID RETENTION).

Preparing and Using: Select plums which look bright and feel soft to the touch; and choose prunes which have been prepared without additives. Sweet, ripe plums are delicious raw; less perfect plums benefit from cooking.

Halve and stone the plums, put them in a heavy-based saucepan or casserole, add some apple juice concentrate (4 tablespoons to 450 g/1 lb plums) and cook gently, with a lid on the pan, or in a covered casserole in the oven, for about 30 minutes, or until tender. Warming flavourings such as cinnamon, ginger, aniseed and fennel can be added. For a plum fool, whizz the cooked plums in a food processor with silken tofu or yogurt.

Prunes are best soaked in cold water for an hour or so, then cooked for 30–45 minutes until tender. A dried fruit salad mix – including prunes, dried apricots, peaches, pears and apple rings – can be prepared like this and makes a delicious pudding. Try flavouring the mixture with different spices, and adding some sliced fresh fruit.

PLUMS, PEACHES, APRICOTS, PRUNES AND DRIED BANANAS

This recipe makes a pleasant breakfast or dessert; it is good for CONSTIPATION. Serves 3.

> *8 prunes*
> *8 dried apricots*
> *3 plums, stoned and sliced*
> *1 peach, stoned and sliced*
> *2 dried bananas, chopped*

Soak half the prunes and dried apricots in water overnight. Next day add the unsoaked prunes and apricots, the plums and peach. Cover with water and simmer for 45 minutes. Eat hot or cold, with the dried bananas added just before serving.

POMEGRANATE *Punica granatum*

Cooling, tonic

Pomegranate – both as a fruit, and in particular, in the form of juice – not only has a very pleasant flavour but also good healing properties. The bright red juice strengthens, cleanses and cools the blood, giving a rosy, fresh complexion. It refreshes and strengthens the heart, fortifies what the Chinese call EMPTY OR WEAK BLOOD (ANAEMIA) and cheers the spirit. It is useful when there is depression alternating with aggression and anger.

The dried and powdered peel is used as a tea for DIARRHOEA and DYSENTERY, and the bark of the root is used to expel intestinal worms, although this is best taken under the guidance of a practitioner.

The best way to obtain pomegranate juice is by using a juicer; if this is not available, purée the flesh in a food processor or liquidiser, then extract the juice by pressing the purée through a sieve.

Preparing and Using: Cut pomegranates in half and remove the red berry-like fruits with a teaspoon. They make a pretty and refreshing garnish for fruit and vegetable salads. Or you could eat the pomegranate from the skin with a pointed grapefruit spoon. The juice can be made into an excellent sorbet if you freeze it, break it up into rough chunks, and whizz it in a food processor.

QUINCE *Malus cotoneus*

Cool, anti-inflammatory

This beautiful golden fruit has a wonderful anti-inflammatory action on the digestive system. Quinces are one of the best remedies for CONSTIPA-TION and at the same time they can reduce DIARRHOEA. They cool and heal ULCERS, ACIDITY, HEARTBURN, GASTRITIS, COLITIS, DIVERTICULITIS and any in-flamed digestive condition. The renowned herbalist Gerard says that quinces are helpful to reduce MENORRHAGIA (EXCESSIVE MENSTRUATION) and for all abdominal pains, whilst Hildegard of Bingen mentions their ability to soothe inflamed joints due to RHEUMATISM.

Preparing and Using: Quinces are not easy to find but they shouldn't be missed. They are best eaten cooked; there is no need to remove the skin, just core them and slice thickly. Cover with water and simmer for

30–40 minutes until tender. If you only have 1 quince, it can be mixed with pears or apples.

COMPOTE OF QUINCES AND FIGS

Prunes, dried apricots, sultanas or raisins can be used instead of the figs, but figs are particularly good for the digestive tract, and are sweet and succulent. This compote tastes delicious, as well as being very soothing and comforting for a delicate overheated stomach, where there is hot, burning INDIGESTION. Serves 2.

> *3–5 figs*
> *1 large quince*
> *3 cloves*
> *a small piece of cinnamon stick*
> *2 teaspoons honey, Barbados sugar or maple syrup (optional)*

Cover the figs with water and soak for a few hours, or overnight. Wash the quince, and cut, unpeeled, into thick slices, discarding the core. Put the quince in a saucepan with the figs, cloves, cinnamon, and sweetening if used. Bring to the boil and boil for 2–3 minutes. Then turn the heat down and cook over a low heat until the fruits are very tender and most of the water has evaporated, leaving a glossy syrup. Remove the cloves and cinnamon stick, and serve hot, warm or cold, with thick Greek yogurt if liked.

RASPBERRY *Rubus idaeus*

Neutral, astringent, tonic

Both the flowers and the leaves of the raspberry plant have been extensively used in the traditional natural medicine of Europe, Arabia, India and China. If sucked slowly, the fruits can improve MOUTH ULCERS and soothe a swollen, SORE THROAT. They are reputed to strengthen the energy of the kidneys and, according to Chinese medicine, this could improve a sore and cold lower back, with general debility and sexual weakness. They have a mildly astringent action for DIARRHOEA and GENITAL DISCHARGES. Dr Valnet considers that raspberries cleanse and strengthen the joints in cases of RHEUMATISM.

Raspberry leaves are used for their astringent qualities as throat gargles, for diarrhoea, discharges and frequent urination.

Raspberry leaf tea has for centuries been thought to help in childbirth if taken during pregnancy. If you want to try it, consult your doctor and ask a herbalist or natural practitioner for specific advice.

Preparing and Using: Wash raspberries carefully and drain in a colander. Serve them plain, or with cream or yogurt. Or push them through a nylon sieve to make a purée and serve with other fresh fruits. This purée can be folded into thick yogurt or cream, or whizzed in a food processor with silken tofu, to make a fool or ice-cream. Sweeten to taste with a little apple juice concentrate.

STRAWBERRY *Fragaria spp.*

Neutral

Strawberries have a general moistening action on the lungs and throat. They are useful for DRY COUGHS, SORE THROATS and for a weak respiratory system generally. They cool an OVERHEATED DIGESTION with symptoms such as GASTRITIS and DIARRHOEA, and, like raspberries, they can improve general vitality.

According to Dr Binet, strawberries cleanse the blood, help the skin and lessen the pain of RHEUMATISM; Dr Gley recommends them for ATHEROSCLEROSIS and for HYPERTENSION (HIGH BLOOD PRESSURE), to keep the circulatory system clear. A tea made from strawberry leaves is prescribed by some European herbalists to help circulation and strengthen the capillaries. Like the fruits, the leaves have a mildly anti-rheumatic action and can also help in diarrhoea.

Note: Some people are allergic to strawberries and after eating them can develop INDIGESTION, swellings and SKIN RASHES.

Preparing and Using: Remove the stems, and halve or quarter the large strawberries so that they are all roughly the same size; rinse in cold water and drain. Sweeten strawberries if you wish by marinating for an hour or so with apple juice concentrate or clear honey; or try them with a raspberry purée.

They are a refreshing addition to summer salads; and you can mix strawberries with peeled and sliced cucumber and chopped mint, with perhaps some curd cheese or cottage cheese, to make a complete light meal. They are also good with avocado: try scooping the flesh out of avocado halves, dicing it and mixing with sliced strawberries, lemon

201

juice and, again, perhaps some chopped mint. Pile the mixture back into the avocado skins and garnish with a sprig of mint.

Strawberries combine well with creams, creamy cheeses and also, for an excellent non-dairy fool, with tofu (see recipe below).

STRAWBERRY AND TOFU WHIZZ

The silken tofu is best for this. If you freeze the strawberries, or use frozen ones, and add them to the tofu without defrosting them the result is a thick, frozen mixture, like a non-dairy ice-cream. It's delicious served with a sauce made by sieving ripe raspberries.

> *450 g/1 lb ripe strawberries, hulled*
> *1 × 275 g/10 oz packet of silken tofu*
> *4 tablespoons clear honey or apple juice concentrate*

Cut the strawberries into even-sized pieces. (For the frozen version of this dish, put the pieces, separated from each other, on a large plate or tray and freeze until firm.) Put the tofu and its liquid in a food processor with the honey or apple juice concentrate. Add the strawberries and whizz until smooth and creamy. If you are using frozen strawberries, the mixture will become icy and thick. Spoon into individual dishes and serve at once.

STRAWBERRIES IN RASPBERRY PURÉE

Serves 4.

> *225 g/8 oz raspberries, washed*
> *apple juice concentrate*
> *450 g/1 lb strawberries, washed, hulled and sliced as necessary*

First purée the raspberries, then push them through a sieve to remove the pips. Sweeten to taste with apple juice concentrate. Then put the strawberries in a serving bowl or 4 individual bowls and pour over the raspberry purée. Serve with some thick Greek yogurt.

WATERMELON *Citrullus lanatus*

Cooling, moist, diuretic

Watermelon is one of the fruits to which people turn for refreshing comfort during the summer months, to cool the body and quench the thirst. It can help SKIN INFLAMMATIONS, SUNBURN, chapped lips, MOUTH ULCERS, FEVERS and all those diseases brought about by excess heat, both internal and external. It is probably the most potent diuretic amongst the fruits and can get rid of OEDEMA (FLUID RETENTION). For this reason, watermelon is also helpful for WEIGHT LOSS.

Preparing and Using: A ripe watermelon should sound hollow, like a drum, when you tap it with your knuckles. It is best served as it is; the seeds can be eaten as well – they add a pleasant crunchiness – or they can be removed if you prefer. A day eating only watermelon is helpful at the beginning of a slimming diet, or from time to time when you feel like a day of cleansing (try and make this a day when you don't have to do anything energetic and can enjoy relaxing).

Watermelon makes an attractive addition to fruit salads. For a healthy yet stunning summer party dessert, cut the top third off a large watermelon, scoop out all the flesh and discard the seeds. Dice the flesh and mix with other summer fruits and perhaps some flowers and aromatic leaves, such as rose petals and borage if available, mint, lemon balm or scented geranium leaves. Vandyke the top of the larger piece of watermelon and cut a slice off the base so that it stands level. If you are feeling artistic, you can write a message on the watermelon or decorate it by scraping designs on it with a canelle knife which you can buy at any kitchen shop.

Food from Animal Sources

It is perfectly possible – and some would say preferable – to live healthily without eating food from animal sources, as long as the diet is properly balanced (as explained on pages 31–8). However, most people like to include some animal products: either just dairy produce and eggs, as part of a vegetarian diet; or meat and fish.

Exponents of natural medicine believe that excessive consumption of animal protein can lead not only to fatty deposits (contributing to heart disease and other illnesses) but also to a general build-up of toxins in the system. In addition, many illnesses such as salmonella poisoning are associated with animal products, and there are the possible long-term risks to human health of BSE ('mad cow' disease).

Since it seems that such conditions may be caused or aggravated by the type of food given to the animals, it is safest to choose organic meat and dairy products. These are also free from possibly harmful chemicals such as antibiotics and hormones. Animal proteins of any kind are best eaten sparingly, more as a condiment and flavouring than the basis of a meal.

DAIRY PRODUCE

In the past, some schools of natural healing, particularly in India, used to recommend milk and other dairy produce for their nourishing properties. They considered these foods – particularly butter – to be moistening and strengthening; especially good for people with brittle bones and dry, crackly joints. They believed that dairy products strengthened all the systems of the body and maintained youthful looks and a good complexion.

There may have been some truth in this. However, the findings of modern research seem to be more in line with the Far Eastern approach which has never emphasised dairy foods. Indeed, evidence now strongly suggests that excessive consumption of such foods can increase cholesterol levels and fat deposits in the body, leading not only to heart disease but to numerous other health problems. Dairy produce also increases mucus production and so can aggravate conditions such as ASTHMA, BRONCHITIS, SINUSITIS and COLDS.

Yogurt is considered to be slightly different from other types of dairy produce; it is easy to digest and does not leave fatty deposits. In fact yogurt has most of the advantages of other dairy products without the disadvantages. Because of the bacteria it contains, yogurt has a beneficial action on the bacteria in our gut. It is particularly helpful when taken after a course of antibiotics because it helps to restore the natural bacteria which the antibiotics have destroyed. If you are on an anti-mucus diet it is best to take even yogurt in moderation. Preferably choose a skimmed variety, and limit the amount to a tub a week. Yogurt is considered to be very cooling, so it is helpful for conditions like hot CYSTITIS and hot INDIGESTION.

Dairy produce can generally be taken in moderation by growing children, or by those who have a strong digestive system and do not suffer from those conditions associated with fat deposits and mucus.

FISH

Of all the animal proteins, fish is probably the healthiest. It is light and easy to digest, and some studies suggest that it could even help to reduce the fat deposits which lead to heart disease.

Oily fish – such as mackerel, salmon, tuna, herrings, sardines and anchovies – are known to contain a fatty acid called Omega 3 which improves the functioning of the cells and helps conditions such as ATHEROSCLEROSIS, HEART AND CIRCULATORY PROBLEMS and SKIN DISEASE, although it should be avoided in diseases where there is a high level of uric acid. It is also best not to eat these fish too often, but to alternate them with other types, as we are not yet completely sure of the long-term effect on a Western population of Omega 3 fatty acids. When eating any fish, it is important to choose varieties caught in unpolluted waters.

According to Chinese medicine, fish is of medium temperature and has some of the properties of other seafoods such as seaweeds (see page 127). It strengthens the general energy of the body and is thus useful for both weak yin and weak yang conditions. It helps to get rid of excessive fluid and dampness in the joints; it also clears the lymphatic system; reduces cysts and swellings, particularly glandular and lymphatic swellings; reduces anal and vaginal discharges; eliminates mucus from the system; and sharpens the memory.

Fish is a good source of protein which, unlike red meat, does not leave toxins or create heat in the system, and therefore does not aggravate hot conditions such as HAEMORRHOIDS (PILES). White fish – like cod, haddock, lemon sole, plaice and whitebait – is helpful during convalescence when the stomach is in a delicate condition and the diet restricted.

EGGS

Eggs are a nourishing food containing good-quality protein as well as many other nutrients such as calcium and phosphorus. The Chinese believed that they could alleviate dryness in the body and improve the quality of the blood. Today it is generally considered that excessive consumption of eggs, like dairy produce, can cause problems with excessive cholesterol, fatty deposits and mucus, although there is some disagreement as to how far this applies to eggs. We think it is best to limit your consumption of eggs to a maximum of 3 per week, produced by free-range hens.

POULTRY

Chicken, turkey, guinea fowl and wild game all contain less saturated fat than pork or red meat and are therefore a more health-giving choice. Turkey has the least saturated fat; duck probably has the most, so it should only be eaten occasionally. Always buy free-range poultry, and remove the skin before eating. The Chinese thought poultry could increase energy in the body and strengthen the blood; however, excessive consumption can block energy in the digestion, creating heaviness and bloating.

BEEF

The Chinese considered beef to be a warm food which strengthened the vital energy and in particular the yang. It also improves the muscle tone and staying-power. However, it is not advised for hot conditions, where there is weak yin or inflammation anywhere in the body, for FEVERS or HYPERTENSION (HIGH BLOOD PRESSURE). In general, beef should be eaten sparingly, mainly during cold weather or periods of physical activity, and always with plenty of vegetables.

LAMB

The properties and uses of lamb are the same as those of beef.

PORK

Because of its high fat content, the Chinese believed that pork could reduce dryness in the body. However, we do not advise the consumption of pork; nor, in particular, products made from it such as ham and salami because of the large quantities of colourings, preservatives and other chemicals which they contain. All these products can increase fat deposits and mucus in the body.

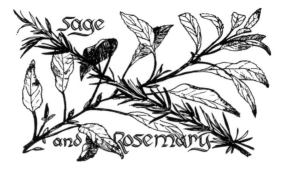

4

The Ailments and How to Treat Them

This chapter tells you how to treat common ailments with natural remedies. The main remedies have already been described fully in Chapter 3, together with details of how to prepare and use them. The ailments are mainly arranged under the 'systems' of the body (rather than alphabetically), to show how the conditions develop and how the body functions as a whole.

If you're not sure what the problem is, you can read a whole section and see if any of the symptoms sound familiar. If you've already identified the specific ailment you can use the Index to find it.

Digestive System

INDIGESTION

Surveys have shown that up to 30 per cent of apparently healthy people suffer from indigestion in varying degrees. The symptoms can include bloating, fullness and tightness in the stomach or chest. In the majority of cases the problem is nervous indigestion, caused by emotional stress, a pressurised lifestyle or nervous tension.

If we eat when we are tense and rushed, our stomach does not have a chance to relax. As a result, food is not properly broken down, assimilated and eliminated. This is SLOW DIGESTION in which pockets of food accumulate in the intestine, leading to putrefaction and inflammation. A person who has this condition feels tense and lacking in vitality, with general tiredness and a feeling of sleepiness in the afternoon. There may be bloating in the abdomen, headaches, mild insomnia and diarrhoea or constipation.

Action taken at this stage can prevent the condition deteriorating into something more serious.

These are the immediate steps you can take:

- Try to eat at regular intervals.
- Before you start eating, check the state of tension in your body. Take a few deep breaths and relax; try to put aside your worries. Allow yourself this time to relax, replenish and regenerate yourself.
- Eat slowly and chew your food well. This helps you to relax, and aids digestion.
- Try to avoid foods which are high in refined starch, such as white bread and white pasta. These can slow your digestion, cause you to feel heavy and lethargic and to put on weight, whilst starving you of minerals and vitamins. Instead, eat wholegrains, balanced with equal quantities of vegetables and pulses. These are easier to digest and supply ample nutrients. Avoid also, as far as possible, white sugar and foods which contain it, and also fried food. For more information on this, see the advice on following a balanced diet (pages 31–8).
- Leave the table feeling light: don't overburden your stomach. This will make you feel heavy and lethargic, and will create gases and distension in your abdomen. If allowed to continue, this condition can create a state of chronic mild indigestion which saps vitality and gives a feeling of being below par. This is defined as stuck or stagnant energy in the abdomen.

STAGNANT ENERGY IN THE DIGESTION always entails distension, swelling, discomfort and soreness. When energy is stagnating in the abdomen it cannot move downwards in the normal way and so comes up and is experienced as indigestion: heartburn, hiccups and belching. The stagnant energy also means that food is digested too slowly, resulting in putrefaction, which is the cause of the distension. When the intestine has to deal with this, it either becomes irritated, resulting in DIARRHOEA (page 210), or it gives up altogether, resulting in CONSTIPATION (page 210).

The advice on following a balanced diet (pages 31–8), and on eating (at the beginning of this section) will help this condition. In addition, the following teas taken frequently, either on their own or mixed together in combinations of two or more, will also be helpful: cardamom, aniseed, fennel, mint, bitter orange peel and camomile. The following spices can be used in cooking: cardamom, fennel, aniseed, mint, basil, cumin, coriander and caraway. Massage your abdomen clockwise three times a week with equal parts of essential oil of orange peel, cardamom and fennel, diluted in a base of massage oil.

Should this condition continue, it will lead to HOT INDIGESTION. The lining of the stomach may eventually become irritated, developing into chronic inflammation or GASTRITIS. When irritation begins it means that stagnant energy is turning into heat. Prolonged stagnation and irritation can cause a hot condition resulting in ULCERS in the stomach or duodenal walls; or an irritated condition like HIATUS HERNIA. In the intestines, this can lead to DIVERTICULITIS, COLITIS, CROHN'S DISEASE, IRRITABLE BOWEL SYNDROME and PILES. The symptoms of heat and fire, or lack of yin energy, in the stomach and intestines, can give symptoms of burning, acidity, red face and eyes; constipation and dry stools; smarting and burning diarrhoea with a strong smell; or bleeding, painful and burning piles. Prolonged stagnation of energy can lead to stagnation of the blood, affecting the circulation, and creating stabbing pains.

In order to improve these conditions, the energy has to be moved and the stomach cooled. This means that all grains should be very well cooked; hot and spicy foods should be avoided, as should alcohol, coffee, white sugar and other over-refined products. The advice on eating a balanced diet (pages 31–8), should be strictly followed. During acute episodes it is best to avoid most dairy products with the exception of a little live yogurt. Follow the ANTI-INFLAMMATION DIET (page 38) and avoid eating too many heavy green vegetables if diarrhoea is a problem. Cabbage, however, is excellent. For many centuries cabbage has been known as a remedy for ULCERS, both external and internal. Only recently researchers have found that cabbage contains vitamin U, which has a strong healing effect on ulcers.

Cabbage juice, extracted with a juicer, or by liquidising cabbage and then pressing it through a sieve or squeezing it in muslin, is a helpful remedy. Dilute a cupful of juice with water and drink half before lunch and half before dinner. It is best to take this lukewarm. If you cannot take that amount at a time, the diluted cabbage juice can be taken in sips throughout the day.

Potatoes also have an anti-inflammatory action but they can be too stodgy. A good way to take them is to add half a raw potato to the cabbage before juicing; or make a soup from cabbage and potatoes (see page 97). Brown rice is excellent; try cooking a little pot barley with the rice – this is very healthy for this condition. Rice water is good, too. To make this, cook the brown rice (or a mixture of rice and barley) with extra water – 3 cups of water to 1 of rice, instead of 2. When the rice is cooked, drain off and drink the extra water slowly during the day.

Pulses are a good source of protein but many people with digestive problems might find that these can exacerbate the condition. The advice

209

on page 137 may help; or you could try tofu (see page 149) which is one of the most digestible forms of pulse and highly nourishing. If you eat meat, it is best to limit this to a little steamed poultry and fish; avoid red meat, and pork and all its derivatives such as ham and salami. Cut bread and pasta to the minimum, since these can aggravate the problem.

DIARRHOEA

If you have diarrhoea, the best food to eat is well-cooked brown rice or millet. A combination of small quantities of grated raw carrot and apple eaten twice a day can be beneficial; have this with the brown rice or millet. Cooked pumpkin, carrots and courgettes (and perhaps a little tofu) are also good. You can eat these all together, in a recipe such as PUMPKIN, COURGETTE AND CARROT SOUP on page 126, or you can just have one of them at each meal, together with the brown rice or millet, and a little tofu if you fancy it. Avoid both cooked and raw green vegetables, and, of the fruits, eat only apples, pears, pawpaw, quinces and raspberries, in moderation.

Drink teas made from camomile, aniseed, rosehip, hibiscus and lemon verbena, varying them as you wish. If you can, get tincture of marshmallow root and tincture of cranesbill root, or bistort, if cranesbill root is not available, mix equal parts of these, and take 20 drops in half a glass of water after meals.

It is also helpful to massage the abdomen clockwise for a few minutes with any of the following essential oils diluted in a base oil, either single or mixed: geranium, camomile, sandalwood, frankincense and lavender.

CONSTIPATION

If there are symptoms of inflammation but with a tendency towards constipation, follow the ANTI-INFLAMMATION DIET on page 38. In addition to the fruits and vegetables suggested, quinces, globe artichokes and fennel are also beneficial, since they are highly anti-inflammatory and have a gentle laxative effect. Combinations of raw and cooked fruits, such as FIGS WITH PRUNES, PEARS AND APPLES (page 186), can be very helpful.

In addition, take 2 teaspoons of psillium seed husks, available from healthfood shops, at night; put the husks in your mouth and then swallow them with some liquid. Continue this treatment until your bowels are back to normal. Try, too, a cup of tea each day made from dried orange peel, fennel and mint. Both these treatments are helpful for all types of constipation.

If the problem is constipation of the hot and dry type, but without accompanying heavy inflammation, you should follow the general guidelines for diet given under INDIGESTION (page 207), being especially careful to avoid refined or semi-refined sugars and any products which contain them. However, you can eat a much wider range of vegetables; in particular, steamed leeks, fennel, onions and wild chicory, cooked globe artichokes and steamed and raw mooli. Pulses are also recommended because of their high fibre content. You can eat vegetables raw as well as cooked, particularly during the summer; and if you dress these with extra virgin olive oil and lemon juice the benefit will be increased.

Another useful remedy is equal parts of tincture of fennel, buckthorn (or cascara if buckthorn is unobtainable), marshmallow root and liquorice. Take 30 drops in half a glass of water before retiring. When the bowel movements are close to normal, omit the buckthorn or cascara from the mixture. You can also take these ingredients as a tea; make this by mixing them together in equal parts, then infuse 1−2 teaspoons in a cup of just-boiled water for 10 minutes.

If the constipation has all the usual feelings of bloating, flatulence and discomfort, but without any symptoms of heat or cold in the body or abdomen, then it is only due to stagnation of energy without heat. In this case, the treatment is the same as that just described, but without the need for extra raw fruit and vegetables.

Both types of constipation, the hot type, and the kind due simply to stagnation of energy, can be helped by massaging the abdomen in a clockwise direction for a few minutes each day with essential oils of sweet fennel and orange peel or grapefruit peel, diluted in the usual way.

If the person suffering from constipation is rather cold and anaemic-looking, the problem may be caused because there is not enough warmth and energy in the body to move the stools. In this case, a more warming and yang diet is needed. This can consist of wholegrains, including some oat bran; the steamed vegetables described above, plus beetroot; fruits in moderation; and pulses. Energising, warming spices like ginger, garlic, and chillies can be used in moderation. The same teas and herbs still apply, too; in addition some tonics, such as ginseng and dang quai are beneficial. These should be taken as recommended by a healthfood shop or herbalist.

COELIAC DISEASE

Coeliac disease, or gluten intolerance, is a condition in which there is diarrhoea and malnutrition due to an allergy to gliadin, a protein in gluten. Gluten is found mainly in wheat and wheat products, such as bread, cakes, flour and pasta; also, in smaller quantities, in oats, barley and rye. You should avoid these grains and all foods containing them, but you can still eat brown rice and rice products, buckwheat and millet, which are both tasty and gluten-free. Read the sections of **The Digestive System** which describe symptoms applying to you, and follow the relevant advice. In this way you will be treating the cause of the problem, which is often chronic inflammation in the intestine.

HAEMORRHOIDS (PILES)

For piles, a cooling and cleansing diet is advised: follow the ANTI-INFLAMMATION DIET (page 38) and the suggestions given for DIARRHOEA (page 210) or CONSTIPATION (page 210). Piles are only an indication of a disorder in the digestive system; and if you treat the cause, rather than the symptom, you should see some improvement.

LIVER AND GALL BLADDER PROBLEMS

The liver is our largest gland. It is situated in the upper right part of the body and weighs 1–2.3 kg. The liver performs many vital functions: removing from the bloodstream toxins and residues from drugs and alcohol; metabolising and storing vital vitamins and iron; assisting in the metabolism of sugars and fats; secreting bile to be stored in the gall bladder and used as part of the digestive process; and balancing the action of many hormones. The liver is the main heat-producing organ in the body; it needs a great deal of energy in order to carry out its many functions and to keep the body warm, energetic and cleansed. Because of this, however, it is easy for the liver, and also the gall bladder, to become congested and overheated.

In traditional natural medicine the main symptoms of an OVERHEATED LIVER AND GALL BLADDER are red eyes and face; 'bursting' headaches; pain or soreness in the right shoulder and side; nausea; dizziness, indigestion and acidity; mainly constipation with dry stools but also sometimes burning diarrhoea; nausea and bitter taste in the mouth; irritability and anger.

To heal this condition, the liver has to be cooled and cleansed. Some of the best foods for this are globe artichokes, cabbage, celery, lettuce and other salad greens, particularly the bitter ones such as dandelion leaf and wild chicory. It is a good idea to have a mixed salad for lunch or supper, including these green leaves, and a dressing of extra virgin olive oil and freshly squeezed lemon juice. Beneficial fruits are bilberries, figs, grapefruits, plums, melon, prunes and pawpaw. Try eating for a month, perhaps for breakfast, as part of a liver-cleansing diet, half a grapefruit and 2–3 plums or prunes, either raw or cooked.

These suggestions should of course be integrated into a balanced diet as described on pages 31–8. It is important to avoid hot spices; fatty and fried foods; refined sugar; all foods and drinks containing chemical additives; alcohol, coffee and red meats. Honey or, especially, molasses, can be taken in moderation as a sweetener. Coffee substitutes such as dandelion and chicory are good, as are teas made from mint, rosehips and hibiscus. Essential oils of rose, geranium and grapefruit can be diluted in the usual way and massaged over the abdomen and liver.

Sometimes liver and gall bladder imbalances manifest with more yin and, in Chinese medical terminology, 'empty or weak blood' symptoms such as nausea; dull headaches; a pale and yellow face; a bitter taste in the mouth; brittle nails and hair; soreness over the right shoulder and side; a feeling of coldness, irritability and depression. For this condition the following fruits and vegetables are recommended, as part of a balanced diet: globe artichokes, celery, wild chicory, dandelion leaves, beetroot, carrots, apples, radishes, grapefruit, plums and prunes. As this is a cooler condition than that of an overheated liver, there does not need to be such an emphasis on raw food and salads, and you can have some warming spices such as thyme, garlic, horseradish, chillies and, most particularly, rosemary. Rosemary can also be taken as a tea, and dandelion and chicory coffee. Tincture or tea of dang quai or centaury are also recommended.

Another condition affecting these two organs is STAGNANT ENERGY IN THE LIVER. This is characterised by soreness over the right side; indigestion with a bloated and sore abdomen; a bitter taste in the mouth; and a sore head. For this, a balanced diet (see pages 31–8), free from coffee, alcohol and fatty food, is recommended. Most fruits and vegetables advised for the two conditions described above can be included, with the addition of orange peel, rosehip, hibiscus and mint teas.

A frequent cause of liver illness is INFECTIOUS HEPATITIS. This condition will respond well to the recommendations given above; choose your diet according to whether the symptoms of heat, cold or stagnation are most dominant. During the time of illness and recovery from hepatitis the liver needs extra supplies of sugars. Most conventional doctors advise a high consumption of white sugar. We strongly disagree, and suggest instead that you get extra glucose by adding maple syrup, honey or raw molasses to your drinks, and increasing your intake of stewed, raw and dry fruits, especially plums and prunes.

The gall bladder, situated underneath the liver, can become inflamed and painful and this is usually due to the presence of GALL STONES. Again, follow the diet for cooling and cleansing the liver (page 213) according to the overall energy balance, whether it is hot and yang, cold and weak, or stagnating. In this case, it is also important to follow the suggestions for cutting down your cholesterol intake (see the ANTI-CHOLESTEROL DIET, page 39). Try also taking, last thing at night, a teaspoonful of virgin olive oil with a few drops of freshly squeezed lemon juice. Continue this for a month and repeat three times in a year. Cornsilk tea, made with the silky strands of maize or sweetcorn, is also recommended. Add to this 15 drops of the tincture of barberry, and take it twice a day. If there are only a few small gall stones this treatment may expel them; it will certainly help you to avoid gall stones. For more about avoiding gall stones, see KIDNEY STONES (page 226).

APPENDICITIS

Acute appendicitis needs urgent medical attention and a doctor should be called without delay. Appendicitis is, however, a condition which often begins with niggling pain and discomfort in the lower abdomen and if the right treatment is given it can be prevented from ever reaching the acute stage. The early warning symptoms are an indication that the digestive system is under stress and that there is inflammation present (see INDIGESTION, page 207). The most helpful diet is the ANTI-INFLAMMA-TION DIET (page 38). After a few days on this, the symptoms will probably have subsided and you can gradually introduce other foods, following the general guidelines given under INDIGESTION (page 208). Essential oils of geranium and sandalwood can be helpful, added to massage oil in the usual way and rubbed gently over the abdomen, but not over the appendix area.

CANDIDIASIS

This is a condition in which the yeast-like fungus, candida albicans, which normally lives in the bowel, over-expands, creating problems in other areas of the body, mainly the genito-urinary and digestive systems, and in the mouth and throat. Although this is a common problem, some modern Western naturopaths, lacking experience and depth of knowledge of traditional diagnosis, tend to diagnose candida far too readily. It is worth bearing in mind that an altered gut flora can be the symptom of a deeper problem and not the cause. The presence of candida albicans can be determined by a stool test and various swabs. In my experience (CDP), such laboratory tests have shown that barely a quarter of patients diagnosed as suffering from candida were in fact carrying the infection; most had other imbalances. It should, however, be mentioned that there is a 20 per cent chance of a stool test for candida resulting in a false negative, so if in doubt, wait a fortnight and then have the test again.

If candida is found to be the problem, you need to go on a YEAST-FREE DIET (see page 38) for a few weeks or months until the symptoms have disappeared and further tests show that you are free from the fungus. The conventional treatment for candida is Niastin, an anti-fungal drug, but there are quite a few natural medicines which could eradicate it. One of these is garlic, especially the purple variety; the dose is 1 clove twice a day with meals. You could also try ti tree essential oil; take 2 drops in water twice a day for 3 weeks, then stop for 7 days before repeating. Massage your abdomen with ti tree essential oil diluted in massage oil in the usual way. Capricin is another remedy which has given excellent results, best taken under qualified medical supervision; and products such as acidophilus, to balance the intestinal flora, are recommended.

FOOD POISONING

Food poisoning is a serious condition and you should seek medical advice as soon as possible. The diarrhoea and vomiting which usually accompany food poisoning are the body's way of eliminating toxins, so they should not be discouraged. It can be helpful to massage the abdomen gently for 1–2 minutes in a clockwise direction using a drop each of essential oils of mint, fennel and rosemary in 1 tablespoon of massage oil. Sips of lemon verbena, camomile or mint tea can help to calm the spasms. Drink plenty of water mixed with a dash of honey or molasses and a pinch of table salt to 600 ml/1 pint. At night take 1–2 teaspoons of psillium husks to help cleanse the intestines. Simply swallow the husks with liquid.

HANGOVER

A hangover, with its symptoms of headache and nausea, sometimes accompanied by vomiting and diarrhoea, is the result of irritation to the stomach lining, liver and kidneys. This irritation needs to be soothed and calmed; teas such as mint, camomile, aniseed and rosehip can be helpful; cabbage juice, very finely chopped cabbage salad (see CABBAGE SALAD FOR A HANGOVER, page 96) often work well, as do pure apple juice, and those first-rate liver-cleansers, prune juice and grapefruit juice, mixed half and half. In deciding which of these remedies to take, let your body be your guide: choose whichever appeals the most. Apart from only drinking in moderation, a hangover can often be avoided by drinking the same quantity of water as of alcohol. For other liver-cleansing remedies see also LIVER AND GALL BLADDER PROBLEMS (page 212).

MOUTH ULCERS

According to traditional medicine, mouth ulcers come about as a result of problems in the digestive system, often fire ascending to the mouth. Read through the descriptions and advice under INDIGESTION (page 207), and follow the dietary suggestions for your energy type. In addition, try rinsing your mouth three times a day with a cup of tea made from raspberry leaves, with 2 drops of essential oil of lavender added.

NAUSEA AND TRAVEL SICKNESS

Nausea, or a feeling of sickness, is a symptom of stagnation of energy in the digestive system. For some reason the energy has become stuck in the stomach and is not moving down. This may be due to stomach or liver problems, but often the underlying cause is nervous tension (see INDIGESTION, page 207).

Nausea is helped by spices which encourage the downward movement of the energy: teas made from ginger, fennel seeds, coriander, orange and mandarin peel and mint. Mint, because of its cooling action, is especially good if there is any feverishness or heat, such as heartburn. If the nausea is due mainly to nerves, camomile and lemon verbena will be helpful, either on their own, or mixed with one or more of the above. A combination like mint, camomile and lemon verbena is cooling (see also the remedies suggested under LIVER AND GALL BLADDER PROBLEMS, page 212).

Travel sickness can be eased by taking ginger, which helps to move the energy down from the stomach. Try taking ginger tea (page 62), or use the tincture; take 10 drops in half a cup of water. Some people find it helpful to suck crystallised or preserved ginger. Mint tea is also good. If the travel sickness is mainly due to nerves, some lemon balm or camomile tea could be helpful. Eating small pieces of dry bread from time to time, whenever you feel sick, can also help.

TEETH AND GUM PROBLEMS

A tooth abscess, with swelling, pus and pain, needs treatment which will kill bacteria and soothe inflammation. Three times a day, apply 2 undiluted drops of essential oil of cloves on a cotton bud; then take a marshmallow leaf, violet leaf or well-washed piece of cabbage leaf and wrap it around the tooth and the abscess; change every 2 hours. If the problem seems acute, do consult a doctor or dentist.

Gum problems are often a sign of digestive complaints and should be treated with the appropriate diet, as described under INDIGESTION, page 207. Receding, red, bleeding gums are a symptom of heat within the digestive system and need a cooling diet; pale, receding gums indicate a cold condition, and will respond to a more warming and yang-raising diet.

HALITOSIS (BAD BREATH)

Halitosis may be caused by gum disease or a tooth abscess, for which local treatment can be given; or it can be a sign of a disturbed digestion (see INDIGESTION, page 207). In either case, rinsing your mouth once or twice a day with half a glass of warm water, to which 1–2 drops of essential oil of fennel or mint have been added, will disinfect your mouth and give a pleasant flavour. Alternatively you could use fennel or mint tea as a mouthwash. Drinking these teas can also be helpful, eliminating putrefaction, helping digestion and leaving a fresh taste in your mouth.

DIABETES AND HYPOGLYCAEMIA

The advice given here is not only for juvenile and mature onset diabetes mellitus but also for non-diabetic sugar imbalances like hypoglycaemia. Many practitioners now consider that hypoglycaemic disturbances, with symptoms such as depression, poor concentration, craving for sweets, and mood swings, are more common than was previously thought. One of the best tests for this is the 6 hours glucose tolerance test which you can ask your doctor to arrange, although you would probably have to pay for it to be done.

If you have this condition, you can help yourself a great deal through diet. Contrary to previous medical opinion, research has now shown that a high-fibre, high-carbohydrate, low-fat diet is most effective in assisting the pancreas to produce insulin which regulates the blood sugar level.

Here are some important pointers:

- Have a diet containing at least 40 per cent wholegrains, but avoid too much bread, even wholewheat.
- Cook 10–20 per cent either rye or buckwheat grains with your brown rice, as they are valuable in helping sugar metabolism.
- Oats, and particularly oat bran, should be eaten regularly.
- All pulses are a good source of high-fibre protein and you should eat them often.
- Try to eat fruits whole rather than as juice, in which the sugar content is more concentrated.
- Avoid dried fruits.
- Try not to binge, as this upsets your whole digestive system and particularly the pancreas.
- Some of the vegetables considered particularly valuable in helping the sugar balance are pumpkin, onions, leeks, garlic, cabbages, wild chicory, nettles, dandelions, artichokes, courgettes and carrots.
- The recommended fruits are apples, wild berries and quinces.
- In addition to a good diet, it is helpful to take supplements of vitamin C, manganese and, particularly, chromium. The following herbs are also useful: jambul seeds, obtainable mainly from homeopathic stores; yarrow; centaury; goat's rue. Try them one at a time, drinking 20–30 drops in water after meals. Make up a massage oil combination, using essential oils of juniper and geranium, and rub this on your upper abdomen for a few minutes 5 times a week. Mild but regular exercise is very important.

Respiratory System

The respiratory system, like the other systems of the body, benefits from a balanced diet as described on pages 31–8; in particular, an ANTI-MUCUS DIET (see page 39).

In addition to the right diet, the respiratory system needs clean air and deep, rhythmic breathing, in order to function well. If you live in a city, try to get away to clear, open countryside as often as possible. When you breathe, practise doing so from your abdomen, breathing in deeply and feeling the sides of your lower ribs expanding. A yoga or T'ai Chi teacher, or even a physiotherapist, could help you to practise this deep breathing, which soon becomes a habit if you do it regularly. Allergies to certain chemicals, animals or house dust can aggravate some respiratory conditions, so if you have a respiratory problem consult your doctor about this possibility, and get some tests done. Needless to say, smoking is not conducive to a healthy respiratory system.

COLDS AND FLU

Colds and flu are classified in Chinese medicine as external attacks of wind. These may be either cold wind, or wind heat.

COLD WIND is when, even if there is some fever, the prevalent symptoms are of coldness and shiveriness, requiring warm drinks and warm surroundings. MISO, OAT AND VEGETABLE SOUP (page 145), thyme and mint or elderflower tea are all helpful, as is the ginger tea, described on page 62, with cinnamon, lemon and honey. Put a few drops of essential oil of eucalyptus on a handkerchief and inhale the aroma, or dilute the oil in massage oil and rub over your forehead, chest and upper back. Take 2–3 garlic capsules each day, and half a teaspoon of horseradish powder mixed with warm water three times a day.

WIND HEAT is when there is a predominance of heat, probably accompanied by sweating, redness, and the need for cold drinks and fresh air. A tea made from mint, or from mint, elderberry leaves and violet leaves, is helpful, as are lemon grass tea, lemon thyme tea or lemon and honey in hot water. Some of the warming spices, such as cinnamon, cloves, ginger and garlic can be taken, even though this is a hot condition. However, these spices should be used in small amounts and in conjunction with other cooling ingredients, such as lemon. You can try essential oil of eucalyptus, as described above for cold wind, as well as oil of mint, used in the same way.

219

EARACHE

Severe earache, especially when accompanied by fever, should always receive prompt medical attention. In Chinese medicine, earache is a condition of either cold wind or wind heat (see COLDS AND FLU, above). In mild cases you can apply a mixture of ti tree and lavender essential oils on a cotton bud to the outer ear; use 3 drops of essential oils in all to a 5 ml teaspoonful of almond or sunflower seed oil. A drop of warmed mullein oil can be put on to cotton wool and put into the ear, or dropped into the ear and plugged with a piece of cotton wool.

THROAT PROBLEMS

This includes conditions such as PHARYNGITIS, TONSILITIS and LARYNGITIS, often accompanied by a cold or flu. The cold or flu should be treated first, according to whether it is a cold wind or wind heat type (see COLDS AND FLU, above). Gargle with sage tea a few times a day, or, for a stronger action, you can add marshmallow leaves or root and agrimony, either as a tea, or in the form of tinctures; a few drops to a glass of water. You can also make a gargle by adding 3 drops of essential oil of clary sage to a glass of warm water, or, alternatively, 1 drop each of clary sage, lavender and ti tree.

COUGHS AND MUCUS, BRONCHITIS, ASTHMA AND SINUSITIS

These are conditions in which there may be inflammation of the air passages and excessive accumulation of mucus which cannot be expelled, causing coughing and varying degrees of difficulty in breathing. If the problem is acute, check first to see if there is a condition of wind heat or cold wind (see COLDS AND FLU, page 219) and deal with that. It is important to realise that no problem to do with excessive phlegm can be resolved satisfactorily without careful attention to diet (see the ANTI-MUCUS DIET, page 39). In particular, avoid the three white substances: white flour, white sugar and milk (and its products).

If the mucus has a yellow, brownish or green colour, the condition is one of mucus and heat. The warming spices, such as ginger, cloves, cinnamon and garlic, which have such good antibiotic and expectorant actions, can still be used, but they need to be cooled. So if you have ginger tea, which is excellent for this condition, add plenty of lemon or lime, and take it with honey, molasses or maple syrup. Have cloves and cinnamon baked with fruits such as apples and pears, and garlic with cooling vegetables or salads.

Other herbs and spices which help expel phlegm are fennel, horse-radish, mustard, oregano, savory, thyme, lemon thyme, marjoram and aniseed. The last two also have a calming action on coughs; all of them, with the exception of lemon thyme and aniseed, need to be combined with cooling ingredients, as described above. Make tea with 2 parts violet leaves and 1 part each of thyme and marjoram; drink 2–3 cups a day, between meals. Massage your chest, upper back and sinus area with essential oils of eucalyptus and mint, mixed into a massage oil, as described on page 45. Follow the ANTI-MUCUS DIET (page 39), including as often as possible in your meals the following foods, which calm heat and soothe the lungs: barley, maize, rice, cabbage, carrots, courgettes, fennel, lettuce, pumpkin, pears, lemons, mandarins, grapefruit, peaches, apricots, quinces, pawpaw and melon.

If the mucus is white and transparent and there is a tendency to shivering and cold symptoms, the condition is one of cold mucus. The herbs and spices mentioned above will again be helpful, but for this condition they do not need to be balanced with cooling items. Follow the ANTI-MUCUS DIET (page 39) but do not eat too many raw vegetables and fruits. Include in your meals hot vegetables such as onions, leeks and radishes, with mustard and horseradish; have baked fruits with plenty of warming spices such as ginger, cinnamon and cloves. Ginger tea with cloves or cinnamon is particularly good, as is the LEEK AND GINGER SOUP on page 113. Violet leaf, mint and thyme tea is also recommended, but this time made with equal quantities of each.

LUNGS

When there is weakness of the respiratory system as well as general weakness and a tendency to catch colds and flu continuously, the problem may be weak chi and yang of the lungs or weak yin of the lungs and dry cough. According to traditional Chinese medicine, the first is basically a cold condition, while the second is a hot condition.

WEAK CHI AND YANG OF THE LUNGS is characterised by pallor, chilliness and a worsening of symptoms in cold weather. Warm and strengthening spices and herbs such as ginger, cinnamon, cloves, garlic, thyme, marjoram, mustard, horseradish, oregano, rosemary, sage and savory are recommended, either as teas or with vegetables, soups and baked fruits. Don't overdo it, though, and overheat your body! You can still eat raw food, particularly during the summer, but preference should be given to warm dishes. Massage your chest with essential oils of ginger, sage or doubly diluted (as described on page 45) oils of thyme and cinnamon, added to a massage oil as usual. The Chinese herb astragalus is highly recommended; it can be mixed with ginseng or taken according to the advice of your healthfood shop or practitioner. You also need to ventilate and strengthen your lungs, preferably in the open air, with exercise and deep breathing.

WEAK YIN OF THE LUNGS AND DRY COUGH is a condition in which heat and dryness are created in the lungs because of lack of yin, or moisture, in the respiratory system. There can be a dry, hacking cough; a pale face with red patches over the cheekbones; night sweats; and a worsening of symptoms in hot weather. A cooling and moist diet is recommended for this condition, with a mixture of cooked and raw fruit and vegetables. Use a variety of salad ingredients; vegetables such as pumpkin, cabbage, courgettes, greens and carrots; and fruits such as melon, pears, peaches, quinces and strawberries. Drink a tea, or take the tinctures, of the following mixed herbs: violet leaves or flowers, borage and plantain. You can also drink rose tea and have ROSE JAM (see page 77) frequently. Massage your chest and upper back with essential oils of geranium or rose, added to massage oil in the usual way.

HAYFEVER

This allergy to pollen causes itchy and watery eyes as well as a sore throat, blocked sinuses and sometimes asthma. Traditional medicine views this condition as a symptom of a deeper energy imbalance in the lungs, creating heat and mucus, or in the liver. Check whether there is heat and inflammation in other parts of your body and refer to the appropriate sections of this book for further information: see COUGHS AND MUCUS (page 220) or LIVER AND GALL BLADDER PROBLEMS (page 212), according to your symptoms. During the danger time, take particular care with your diet (see the ANTI-MUCUS DIET on page 39), avoiding hot spices, red meat and alcohol in addition to those foods mentioned, since these aggravate the heat and inflammation present in hayfever. About three weeks before the season, start taking some homeopathic pollen.

Urinary System

CYSTITIS

Before discussing the treatment of cystitis, two practical matters need to be clarified regarding the advice you may be given. Firstly, particularly in Western countries where toilet paper is the main way of cleaning oneself after a bowel movement, the usual advice given for avoiding cystitis is to wipe oneself away from the genitals. This is because bacteria from the bowel can enter the genitals, especially in women. This advice on its own, however, is fairly useless because even if the bacteria are wiped in the other direction, they do not lose their way that easily! They soon seek out the warm and moist surroundings of the genitals. In order to avoid this possibility, it is necessary, after using toilet paper, to wash around the anus and perineum with warm water and a neutral soap.

The second point concerns the advice commonly given to take bicarbonate of soda in order to alkalise the urine. Try to avoid doing this. The effect is only temporary and in a second stage the acidity of the urine increases to balance the excessive alkaline intake, creating a vicious circle. Taking barley water (page 154) and cornsilk tea and following the related recommendations should improve your condition greatly.

Like many conditions, cystitis may be of the hot type or the cold type, and it is treated accordingly. COLD CYSTITIS often affects women. It comes about through getting cold in the bladder, either through wearing inadequate clothing or through having too much cold food or drink. There is a tendency to feel cold and shivery, with cramp-like pains in the bladder and frequent urination. The urine is usually clear or slightly clouded.

This condition is relieved by warmth: warm clothes, a warm environment and warm foods. Soups and teas with warming spices such as ginger and thyme are good; try CARROT, COURGETTE, THYME AND GINGER SOUP (page 102), or sauté these vegetables with thyme and ginger. Bearberry leaf tea taken twice a day can also be helpful. In addition, try massaging the bladder area gently with warm oil with essential oils of lavender and eucalyptus added in equal parts. If you start this treatment as soon as the symptoms begin, the discomfort should soon stop.

HOT CYSTITIS, where there is inflammation in the bladder, is far more common. It can take the form not only of cystitis but also NON-SPECIFIC URETHRITIS (NSU) and THRUSH. The main symptoms are frequent, painful and burning urination possibly even with occasional bleeding. The

223

urine is dark and heavily clouded with an unpleasant smell; and there may be extreme discomfort, sometimes lasting many days or even weeks. Some of the causes of this condition are excessive consumption of hot spices, fatty and fried food, coffee and alcohol; prolonged use of antibiotics altering the flora of the gut or vagina; micro-organisms transmitted through sexual intercourse or from the bowel as a result of poor hygiene; or allergies to a variety of chemical irritants. Any of these reactions can be exacerbated by following incorrect advice.

In treating this condition it is important at the outset to find out, through the proper tests, whether any organisms are present. If so, your doctor will prescribe some antibiotics. Should these fail to work, or if the tests show that you have a non-microbial infection, you can try the following suggestions:

- Avoid all the foods and drinks mentioned above; also red meat, sugar and all products containing it.
- Follow the ANTI-INFLAMMATION DIET (page 38), consisting mainly of wholegrains such as brown rice and barley, and vegetables, especially courgettes, carrots, pumpkin and cabbage. Have the COURGETTE, POTATO AND ONION SOUP (page 105).
- Avoid unripe and acidic fruits such as citrus. The best fruits are apples, pears, pawpaw and melon.
- Drink liberal amounts of barley water, made as on page 154 but with only a few drops of lemon.
- Take 15 drops of propolis tincture twice a day between meals.
- You can also take 2 drops of essential oil of lavender or ti tree in a little water, especially if there is an infection, but do not continue this treatment for more than a few days without taking expert advice.
- Ask your herbalist or healthfood shop to mix for you the following herbs or tinctures in equal amounts: marshmallow root, bearberry and cornsilk. Take the herbs as a decoction twice a day, or the tincture in water, also twice a day, always between meals.

KIDNEYS

According to Chinese medicine, kidney problems and chronic kidney-adrenal metabolic weaknesses are caused by energy imbalances. These are weak yang of the kidneys and weak yin of the kidneys.

In WEAK YANG OF THE KIDNEYS, the person feels tired and is quickly fatigued. They look pale and feel the cold easily. They have weak sexual desire and frequently pass a large volume of pale urine. They might have lower back pain, especially around the kidney area. They should choose warming, yang food, eating raw and yin food only in moderation. The diet should consist mainly of wholegrains, sautéed vegetables, particularly onions, leeks, carrots and celery (see page 26), with warming spices such as garlic, cinnamon, ginger, rosemary, thyme, oregano, savory and sage. MISO, OAT AND VEGETABLE SOUP (page 145) is recommended. Chinese tonics like ginseng and, particularly, schizandra are beneficial: ask your practitioner or healthfood shop to advise you on dosage. Massage your back around the kidney area with essential oils of rosemary, ginger or juniper, added to a carrier oil.

When the problem is WEAK YIN OF THE KIDNEYS, the person complains of lower back pain and general weakness. The problem here is that there is too little yin moisture in the system to balance the fire of the yang. The person may be pale except for redness around the cheekbones. They may complain of night sweats and hot feet and hands, especially in bed. They have a frequent urge to urinate but they only pass small quantities of dark and red urine.

Often, because of their lassitude, these people are wrongly diagnosed as being too yin and are advised to eat a yang diet with high sodium items like miso and tamari. Not only will this fail to improve their condition, it will probably make it worse. The right diet is one based on wholegrains, vegetables and pulses, with the addition of cool, raw and moist food. Of the pulses and pulse products, tofu and mung beans are recommended. Melon, pineapple, pawpaw, bilberries, blackcurrants and peaches help to cool heat in the kidneys and cleanse the urine. Hot spices should be avoided, as well as salty foods, alcohol and coffee. The Chinese tonics rehmania or licium are beneficial; ask your healthfood shop or practitioner for products and dosages.

Conflicting advice is often given about how much liquid you should drink when you have urinary or kidney problems. Some practitioners advise drinking as much as possible throughout the day to flush out the kidneys and bladder; others, including the macrobiotic school, say that intake should be restricted and drinks should be taken warm. When the urinary tract is inflamed and infected it is reasonable to increase the intake of fresh water, either filtered or mineral. But it is important to ensure that the water does not contain high levels of either sodium or calcium (see page 32).

Kidney inflammation and infection includes NEPHRITIS, PYELONEPHRITIS and GLOMERULONEPHRITIS. It is important to remember that we are dealing here with mild states of inflammation, although more serious conditions might also benefit from the following treatment in conjunction with correct medical attention. One must avoid taxing the kidneys, especially during the acute phase, so it is best not to eat salt, animal proteins (with the exception of white fish), or dairy products (except for a little yogurt). Do not eat take-aways or tinned food; avoid asparagus and acid foods such as citrus fruits, vinegar and pickles. Sugar encourages the growth of bacteria and so should be avoided, including honey.

Drink more water than usual but filter it, or, if it is bottled mineral water, make sure that it does not have a high sodium content (see page 32). Eat frequently a combination of 30 per cent potato and 70 per cent courgettes; together they have a very good anti-inflammatory action on the kidneys. Pumpkin, carrots, lettuce and cabbage are also beneficial, as are well-cooked grains, especially sweetcorn and barley, but not wheat flour or products made from it. You can have baked or boiled apples, pears and quinces, and raw, ripe pawpaw. Drink tea made from cornsilk twice a day, and one cup of pure dandelion coffee each day. Tinctures of barberry and marshmallow root can be taken: mix them together in equal parts and take 20 drops in a glass of water twice a day. You can apply to the kidney area some essential oils of lavender, geranium or sandalwood, added to massage oil in the usual way.

KIDNEY STONES can be found in the kidneys, ureter and bladder. The first stage in treating them is to ascertain what has caused them and the substance from which they have formed. Stagnation, or a backward flow of urine when the bladder is not emptying properly, can make one vulnerable to stones and urinary infections.

For this condition, you need to eat diuretic foods, as advised under OEDEMA (see below). If the stones are composed of calcium, you should exclude from your diet all dairy products and water with a high calcium content. Stones formed from oxalic acid mean that tea, coffee, chocolate, rhubarb, peanuts, spinach, beetroot, tomatoes and strawberries should be avoided. Urate stones show that you should stop eating prurine-rich foods like asparagus, red meats, pork, offal, tea, coffee, chocolate, cocoa, cola drinks, sardines, anchovies, whitebait, sprats, mussels, scallops, fish roe, partridge and guinea fowl, as well as alcohol. Eat foods which will promote urination and cleanse the kidneys, as advised under OEDEMA.

If the stones are quite small sometimes the diet suggested, together with a high fluid intake (preferably mineral water with a low calcium content) will get rid of them. Tincture or tea of barberry mixed with cornsilk and taken 2–3 times a day, is also very useful. To lessen the pain when the stone is being expelled, you can take the homeopathic remedy, Silica 6, every half hour until the symptoms ease.

OEDEMA (SWELLING DUE TO WATER RETENTION)

This advice is not so much for the oedema caused by complex diseases of the heart and liver, but for the type caused by what natural medicine views as a mild insufficiency of kidney energy. Cucumber, globe artichokes, asparagus, celery, leeks and parsley are the best vegetables for this condition; also various seaweeds. Corn has a slight diuretic action. Watermelon is probably the strongest diuretic fruit; other useful ones are pineapple, grapefruit, bilberries, peaches and melon. Try to avoid salt and all salty foods, such as smoked meat and fish. The following teas are very useful: rosehip, hibiscus, fennel, dandelion root, aniseed and cornsilk. Tinctures of dandelion, fennel, aniseed and cornsilk can also be taken. Mix them together in equal parts and take 20 drops twice a day in a glass of water between meals.

Reproductive System

PELVIC INFLAMMATORY DISEASE (PID)

Pelvic inflammatory disease, or PID, is the general name given to an internal infection in a woman's reproductive system, and it requires prompt medical attention. Diet, herbs and essential oils can, however, assist the treatment. PID could involve SALPINGITIS (inflammation of the fallopian tubes), PELVIC ABSCESS, ENDOMETRITIS (inflammation of the mucus lining of the womb) or VAGINITIS (inflammation of the vagina). If any of these are due to bacterial infection, as is often the case, some of the advice given under CYSTITIS (page 223) may be helpful.

Since, according to traditional Chinese medicine, any inflammation means that there is too much heat in the body, PID can be helped firstly by eating a more cooling and balanced diet. Baked or boiled fruits, particularly quinces (see COMPOTE OF QUINCES AND FIGS, page 200), are recommended, but do not drink too many fruit juices, especially orange. During the attack, keep clear of alcohol, coffee, sugar, hot spices, fried and fatty food, additives and red meats, because all these can increase the inflammation and worsen the PID (see the ANTI-INFLAMMATION DIET on page 38). In addition, try taking a mixture of equal parts of tinctures of calendula (marigold), marshmallow root, cornsilk and plantain. You can also very gently apply, not massage, the following essential oil combination on the abdomen: lavender, geranium and, if possible, camomile (which is expensive).

PREMENSTRUAL TENSION OR SYNDROME (PMT OR PMS)

Chinese medicine sees this as hyperactivity of the liver and gall bladder, creating irritability, sore breasts, headaches and bloating; and hypo-activity of the pancreas, creating depression, poor concentration, craving for sweets, and mood swings. Research done in England has shown that after a 6 hour glucose tolerance test many women suffering from PMT were found to have hypoglycaemia. Therefore what is needed is a diet which calms the liver and strengthens the pancreas, especially from mid-cycle till the beginning of the period.

Foods which irritate the liver, like hot spices, fatty and fried foods, alcohol, additives and coffee, should be avoided or eaten only in very moderate quantities, as should red meat. A balanced diet should be followed as described on pages 31–8 (see also the dietary advice under LIVER AND GALL BLADDER PROBLEMS, page 212). Remember that sugar, particularly white sugar, is detrimental to the pancreas; you can substitute natural sweeteners for sugar (see page 36), but again only in very moderate quantities because they, too, can deliver too much sugar to the pancreas. Also, be extremely sparing in your intake of refined grains in foods like white bread, pasta and white rice.

Many women with PMT have reported beneficial effects from taking supplements containing evening primrose; ask your practitioner or local healthfood shop about these. Also, you may find it helpful to take the following herbal mixture twice a day from 10 days prior to the period: mix together equal parts of tinctures of blue cohosh, cramp bark, camomile, lemon balm and calendula (marigold); take 20–30 drops in half a glass of water a couple of hours before or after meals.

Have baths with relaxing essential oils such as lavender, geranium, orange peel, mandarin peel, camomile and aniseed: choose the ones you like. Many women have also benefited greatly from gentle exercise and relaxation or meditation techniques (see pages 269–72).

DYSMENORRHOEA (PAINFUL PERIODS)

The advice given under PMT also applies to this condition. In addition, you could try gently massaging your abdomen with essential oils of aniseed, lavender and, if possible, camomile (which is expensive). Start doing this once a day at least 3 days before a period.

AMENORRHOEA (LACK OF PERIODS)

If your periods have recently ceased, first make sure that there is no other cause such as pregnancy. Chronic amenorrhoea for no apparent reason could be due to what the Chinese call a 'weakness of blood'. In this case the woman looks and feels quite anaemic (see page 30). If, in addition, there is a general feeling of coldness with weak and cold limbs, then there is a lack of yang energy (see page 26) and you need to adjust your diet to help correct the basic imbalance.

Try drinking a tea or tincture of mugwort or sage. Take this once a day for 3 weeks, then stop for a week; try the treatment again for 3 more weeks at the most. Also make up an essential oil massage combination with sage and rosemary; massage this gently over your abdomen in a clockwise direction for about 3 minutes every day. Stop using the herbs and oils when a period starts and repeat the treatment only after 3 weeks. Do not continue this treatment for more than 3 months. We must categorically state that this is a very mild form of treatment for amenorrhoea. It cannot, and should not in any way, be used to produce an abortion.

MENORRHAGIA (EXCESSIVE MENSTRUATION)

First make sure that there is no natural cause, such as womb fibroids or polyps. According to Chinese medicine, one of the likely causes is hyperactivity and heat of the liver and gall bladder, and hypoactivity of the pancreas; the diet and advice given for PMT (see above) can also help this condition. Try, too, a tea or tincture of this combination: lady's mantle, shepherd's purse and calendula (marigold). Take the mixture twice a day from 10 days before and then during your period. During this time, also apply essential oils of geranium and sandalwood, mixed with a massage oil, just to your lower abdomen. Do not repeat these treatments for more than three cycles; if symptoms persist, seek medical advice.

LEUCORRHOEA (EXCESSIVE VAGINAL DISCHARGE)

If this is due to some form of PELVIC INFLAMMATORY DISEASE or infection, read the advice on page 227 and under CYSTITIS on page 223.

Sometimes, however, leucorrhoea is present without any obvious cause. If the discharge is rather white, transparent and odourless, it is due to cold and weak yang energy in the system. Follow the advice on page 26 for a yang-strengthening diet. Massage your lower abdomen with essential oils of either ginger or rosemary. If the discharge is yellowish and rather smelly, there is an excess of mucus and heat in the lower abdomen; follow the advice for hot mucus (page 30) and the ANTI-INFLAMMATION DIET on page 38.

In either case, you can try douching about twice a week with 1 teaspoon of tincture of either bistort or cranesbill root, and 1 drop each of essential oils of lavender and sandalwood, in 600 ml/1 pint of lukewarm water. Continue until the condition improves. You can also massage the lower abdomen daily with a combination of the same essential oils.

THRUSH (CANDIDA)

This condition is caused by the yeast-like fungus, candida albicans, affecting the vaginal area, and the treatment is the same as that described for CANDIDIASIS (see page 215). To reduce the discomfort and itchiness you can use the douche described above for LEUCORRHOEA; also try soaking tampons in live yogurt and inserting for a few hours at a time.

NON-SPECIFIC URETHRITIS (NSU)

This condition should be promptly treated by a medical practitioner. For helpful natural remedies, see under CYSTITIS (page 223).

FIBROIDS AND CYSTS

Because fibroids and cysts are also a type of growth, you may find it helpful to follow some of the advice in the section on **Cancer** (pages 240–3).

MENOPAUSE

Simply some of the symptoms which can make this time uncomfortable are hot flushes, night sweats, palpitations, anxiety, and dryness, particularly vaginal. These are seen in Chinese medicine as a weakening of the yin energy and a rising of the yang energy, particularly in the liver. Read the advice under OVERHEATED LIVER (page 231), and also the section on **The Heart and Circulatory System** (pages 243–6).

Add a few drops of essential oils of sage and geranium to your bath, and give yourself a massage with these oils often; on your feet and hands, over your shoulders, down your spine, abdomen and legs. Essential oil of rose is also beneficial and is a lovely treat, but it is one of the most expensive oils. The following, taken as teas or tinctures, can be quite good for strengthening the yin: roses, violets, rehmania, sage and licium. You can just take one, or mix up to three of them. For anxiety, palpitations and insomnia, you can try taking any two of the following, as tea or tinctures: passiflora, hawthorn tops, camomile and lemon verbena. These are best taken last thing at night.

IMPOTENCE, FRIGIDITY AND STERILITY

Problems related to sex and reproduction are definitely exacerbated by emotional and physical tension, and can improve with counselling, relaxation, meditation and gentle exercise (see pages 269–72). It is important for both partners to be patient and sympathetic to each other's needs. If there are no major physical problems behind these conditions, natural medicine and diet can also help.

In Chinese medicine the kidney-adrenal area is considered to be very important for sexual energy and reproduction. Often a weakness in this area is associated with either WEAK YIN or WEAK YANG OF THE KIDNEYS (see page 224).

Infertility and lack of sexual energy caused by a weak yin nature, particularly in a woman, can be helped by taking royal jelly, rose tea or tincture, and ROSE JAM (see page 77). Vitamin E is also helpful for both weak yin and weak yang of the kidneys.

MASTITIS (INFLAMMATION OF THE BREAST)

In its acute form, mastitis mainly affects breast-feeding mothers, although it has been estimated that 15–20 per cent of non-nursing women also have a degree of chronic mastitis.

Acute mastitis in nursing mothers can be due to hormonal changes or to a local bacterial infection. This is a condition which needs prompt medical attention and it is usually treated with antibiotics, particularly if the cause is bacterial. Treatment with essential oils and herbs is not advisable because these could affect the baby. However, if the symptoms persist after taking the antibiotics, it might be worth consulting a homeopath. In any case, you can greatly help the condition by avoiding all foods which increase pain and inflammation in the body: that is, sugar, and all products which contain it; red meat; fried food and fatty sauces; alcohol; hot spices and curries; and coffee.

In non-acute, chronic mastitis, inflammation may be the main problem, or it might be caused by quite painful cysts. In the case of cysts, the fluid may need to be drawn off. In either case, do seek medical advice, and at the same time follow a healthy diet, avoiding the foods mentioned above and bearing in mind the advice given in the ANTI-INFLAMMATION DIET (page 38). If inflammation is the main problem, you can drink a combination of calendula (marigold) and marshmallow root, either as a tincture or a tea.

If the problem is due to cysts, you could also follow the recommendations given in the section on **Cancer** (pages 240–3), merely because in traditional medicine similar advice applies to all kinds of growths. For both these types of chronic mastitis, essential oils of lavender, geranium and frankincense can be helpful. Mix them with a massage oil and apply to the breast once every 24 hours, either during the day or at night.

Skin and Hair

ACNE AND OTHER SKIN PROBLEMS

Many common skin complaints, such as ACNE, ECZEMA, ABSCESSES, HIVES (NETTLE RASH) and PSORIASIS, are, according to traditional medicine, created by toxins accumulating in the blood. This may be due to weak functioning of one of the organs of elimination, such as the liver, colon, lungs or kidneys. The accumulation of toxins leads to heat in the blood which then affects the skin.

If the spot or sore patch is mostly dry, red and inflamed, it is mainly due to heat and lack of yin energy in the body. Look under **The Digestive System** (page 207–18) and check if you are suffering from any of the conditions described, particularly one of the hot ones. Faulty digestion, especially CONSTIPATION (see page 210) is often at the root of a poor skin condition; a balanced diet with a tendency to cooling and yin-strengthening food (see page 26) is needed. Once the underlying digestive condition has been corrected, the skin will improve. You could also add to your bath a few drops of the following essential oils: lavender, geranium, and rose if you can afford it. In addition, you can make a massage oil with these essential oils and apply it to your skin after a bath or shower.

You might like to try the following herbal combination, to cleanse and cool your blood. Mix together rehmania root, heartsease, pellitory of the wall and dandelion root. Add 1 tablespoon of the mixture to 1 litre/1¾ pints water and bring to the boil over a low heat. Then take off the heat and allow to cool, covered, for 20 minutes. Filter and drink at least 1 hour before or after meals for a period of 24 hours. Alternatively, you can use the tinctures of these herbs. In this case, mix the tinctures together in equal proportions, then put 1 tablespoon of the mixture into 1 litre/1¾ pints water and drink over 24 hours, again, at least an hour before or after meals.

If the skin tends to come out in abscesses, spots or boils which are inflamed and pussy, the complaint is due to hot mucus in the system. For this, follow the ANTI-MUCUS DIET on page 39, and try the following herbal mixture: echinacea, plantain, cleavers and heartsease. Prepare and take this as described above. You could also put a few drops of essential oils of lavender, frankincense and sandalwood in your bath; and make a massage oil with the same essential oils, to be applied daily to the affected areas.

Sometimes the body cannot cure itself of the skin problem because the blood is weak or anaemic. In this case, as well as having any of the spots or sore patches described above, the person will look pale and feel tired, with weak nails and brittle hair. Follow the advice given for EMPTY OR WEAK BLOOD (see page 30).

To keep your skin in good condition, try gently massaging your face once or twice a day with a teaspoon of almond oil mixed with 1 drop of essential oil: rose or geranium for a dry or normal skin; lavender or jasmine for an oily skin; and either geranium or lavender for a combination skin. An older skin benefits from the addition of a little wheatgerm oil; break open a wheatgerm capsule and add the contents to the massage oil mixture. If you have an oily skin, finish by gently cleaning off the oil with a piece of cottonwool wrung out in warm water, or with a little orange flower water. For a dry or normal skin, you can use rosewater as a toner.

ITCHING

PRURITIS, ANII AND VULVAE, all itchy conditions, are symptoms of a stressed and overheated liver, or what in Chinese medicine is known as liver fire, or heat in the stomach, or large intestine. The liver needs to be cooled and cleansed: see the section on **The Digestive System** (pages 207–18), and the advice given under LIVER AND GALL BLADDER PROBLEMS (page 212). You can use the essential oil combinations described under ACNE AND OTHER SKIN PROBLEMS in the bath, or add them to a massage oil and apply externally. Calendula (marigold) ointment, from healthfood shops, is also recommended.

WARTS

This viral infection of the skin is best treated by applying calendula (marigold) ointment, from healthfood shops, twice a day. Also try to get essential oil of tagetes (African marigold). Put a drop of essential oil of tagetes on the wart, and then apply the calendula ointment as well. In addition, take one homeopathic Thuja 6 tablet every morning and evening. Continue this treatment for about 3 weeks; then, if unsuccessful, consult your practitioner. While following this treatment try to keep a balanced diet which suits your body type (see **The Basic Conditions**, pages 25–30).

HERPES SIMPLEX (COLD SORES)

Herpes simplex is a common infectious virus which can cause small blisters, commonly called cold sores, usually on the lips, but also on other parts of the face and body, including the genitals. During an attack, try to avoid foods containing arginine, an amino acid which can trigger an eruption. These include wheat and wheat products, such as bread, pasta and biscuits; carob, chocolate, gelatine, coconut, oats, peanuts and soya beans. The following foods can also worsen an attack: red meats, sugar, coffee, fried food and hot spices.

Another amino acid, lysine, is very effective in combating the virus and is found in most fruit and vegetables as well as beans and bean-sprouts, fish, lamb, chicken, milk, cheese and brewer's yeast. You can buy lysine capsules from healthfood shops; take 1.5 g daily while the virus is active. For external application, add 1 drop each of essential oils of ti tree, lavender and geranium to 1 tablespoon of a massage oil such as almond oil, or a pure vegetable face cream. Apply this to the cold sore

234

twice a day. Remember that even after the sore disappears the area could still be contagious for another 3 days. Always seek prompt medical attention for cold sores near the eyes.

For genital herpes, which develops from the virus herpes simplex II, follow the same diet and treatment, of course avoiding sexual contact when the sores are active. In addition, have baths with the essential oils added, and wear loose cotton underwear.

HERPES ZOSTER (SHINGLES)

The virus which causes this painful condition can lie dormant for many years. According to Chinese medicine, it is triggered by heat in the system, particularly in the liver, so you should follow the diet recommended for OVERHEATED LIVER (page 212). To treat the rash directly, first apply an ointment containing calendula (marigold) and hypericum; you can get this from your local healthfood shop; in England it is usually sold under the name Hypercal. Put this on the sores (don't massage them at all because this could spread the infection); then apply the ointment prescribed above for herpes simplex.

BRUISES

Very gently apply homeopathic arnica ointment directly on to the bruise, or use arnica tincture, sprinkling it on to a pad of cottonwool or soft cloth wrung out in cold water, and holding it or bandaging it in place. Only use this treatment if there are no cuts, because arnica should not enter the bloodstream. An alternative is to soak cottonwool or a piece of soft cloth in witch hazel, which you can buy at any chemist. A few drops of essential oil of lavender can be applied to the bruise to help reduce pain, and RESCUE REMEDY (see page 269) can be given for shock.

BURNS

After putting the burn under cold running water, three very effective treatments for minor burns are essential oil of lavender, Bach rescue remedy, both applied neat, and the burn ointment which you can buy from healthfood shops and herbalists. If you put any of these on immediately, they will prevent a blister forming: keep some in the kitchen! More serious burns of course need urgent medical attention but a good first aid measure is to pour undiluted essential oil of lavender on to clean gauze and put this over the burn. For shock, give RESCUE REMEDY (see page 236) which can be dropped straight on to the tongue, or added to a small amount of water and taken in small sips.

HAIR LOSS, BALDING AND DANDRUFF

If hair loss is the problem, firstly make sure from your general practitioner that it is not due to some medication you have taken, such as hormones, antibiotics or steroids, or to a local infection. Check also that you are not suffering from glandular imbalance. Balding can often start at an early age, especially in men; it may be an inherited tendency which is then aggravated by stress and illness.

Traditional medicine considers that, particularly in this condition, the internal treatment is as important as the external, if not more so. Any imbalances of the body functions can result in a weakness which produces hair loss. The condition which the Chinese refer to as weak blood, or anaemia, can mean that the hair does not receive enough nourishment; whereas too much toxicity and fire rising to the head can make the scalp sore and burn out the hair. Conversely, if the yang is too weak, the energy will not rise and the hair will look dull and lifeless. So check first to see if you have any of the energy imbalances mentioned in **The Basic Conditions** (pages 25–30). Also, if you feel that you have any problems in any particular system of your body, look under the relevant heading. In any case, eat millet often, at least 2–3 times a week; and try taking the vitamin combinations for strengthening the hair, available from healthfood shops.

For external treatment there are some remedies you can try but we can't promise any miracles! Ask your herbalist to prepare the following mixture: 40g/1½ oz nettles; 25 g/1 oz sage and 15 g/½ oz each of lavender and rosemary. Mix the ingredients very well and put 1 heaped tablespoon into 300 ml/½ pint water. Bring to the boil, then remove from the heat and let it sit, well covered, for at least 3 hours. Add 1 drop each of the following essential oils: sage, lavender and rosemary. Filter the mixture, then pour it into a jar and keep it in the fridge. Every day, after washing your hands thoroughly, apply some of the liquid to your scalp with the tips of your fingers. When you wash your hair put the water for the final rinse in a large jug or bucket and add 4 tablespoons of the mixture to it. Make up a fresh batch of the lotion every week.

Another rather messy treatment that you might like to try is to take 2 handfuls of watercress, or a mixture of watercress and fresh nettles if available, and whizz them to a purée in a liquidiser or food processor. Spread this over your scalp and leave for 2 hours before washing.

Joints and Bones

JOINT PROBLEMS

Joint problems include conditions such as RHEUMATOID ARTHRITIS, RHEU-MATISM, BURSITIS (HOUSEMAID'S KNEE OR TENNIS ELBOW) and GOUT, where there is swelling, deformation and inflammation. Conventional medicine still has no answer as to the cause of most joint problems, and the treatment is sometimes very toxic. Traditional schools of naturopathy in the West mainly ascribe these problems to toxic accumulation in the joints due to unhealthy diet and poor digestion and elimination. Chinese medicine sees the cause as an energy imbalance, and classifies joint problems as hot or cold, according to the symptoms.

HOT RHEUMATISM is when the joints are red, dry and painful, with the symptoms becoming more intense during hot and humid weather; COLD RHEUMATISM is the type with cramp-like pains like a claw tightening around the joint, and the symptoms are worse in cold and humid weather. Chinese medicine also emphasises the fact that rheumatism is very often created by a damp or humid environment. This may be due to the weather or to damp living conditions, perhaps through work which entails prolonged contact with water, as in kitchens or flower shops. It can also be caused by eating too many fatty or fried foods, alcohol, meats, raw vegetables and fruits containing a large percentage of moisture. Dampness can occur in both hot and cold types of rheumatism; if it is present there will always be swelling as well as the other symptoms.

Not only the diagnosis, but also the approach of traditional medicine and conventional medicine towards these problems is very different. Conventional medicine concentrates on powerful chemicals which can temporarily alleviate the symptoms, but possibly at the risk of increasing toxicity in the system, thus aggravating the condition in the joints. Traditional medicine concentrates on removing the toxins in the joints through a cleansing diet, and on removing the environmental conditions which aggravate the condition.

Many thousands of people have experienced improvement in their condition through changing their eating habits. Read the advice on eating a balanced diet (pages 31–8), and look also at the section on

The Basic Conditions (pages 25–30), adding to your diet the foods recommended for your emotional and body type. Avoid those foods which can aggravate joint conditions: citrus fruits, spinach, chocolate, coffee, red meat, pork, tomatoes, sugar, grains and alcohol. Many patients have also found great relief through following a food-combining diet: that is, eating protein foods (eggs, cheese, milk, meat and fish) and starch foods (bread, potatoes, pasta and cereals) at separate meals; and not mixing acid fruits (that is, all fruits except the very sweet, starchy ones, like bananas, dried and fresh figs, pawpaw, ripe sweet pears, raisins and dates) with starch meals. Especially at the beginning of the illness, and between acute periods, try to practise mild exercises to keep the joints flexible; some simple yoga techniques can be helpful (see page 270). Gentle osteopathic treatment to stretch the joints through articulatory techniques is also recommended.

It is worth checking whether your general attitude to life is contributing to the problem. Stiff and painful joints may show a fear of moving forward, or a stiffness and rigidity of outlook. Examine yourself very carefully for any fears or beliefs which may also be exacerbating the condition. Visualise yourself frequently being free from pain and with your body perfectly whole and healthy; it has happened to others, and it can happen to you. See the section on **Relaxation, Meditation and Visualisation** in the chapter on 'Helping the Healing Process' (pages 271–2).

COLD JOINT PROBLEMS

With this type of problem, there may be a general feeling of coldness and a weakness of yang energy, as well as the symptoms already described. The condition will be relieved by warmth from the sun, a heating pad or electric blanket, warming linament, or moxibustion (a treatment in which a burning stick is held just above the painful area or over an acupuncture point). You can also make a massage oil with essential oils of either ginger or rosemary to warm and alleviate the arthritis; add essential oil of lavender to soothe the pain and swelling. Avoid raw food and very moist fruits like pineapple, peaches and grapes, especially in cold weather; follow a more warming and yang-raising diet (see page 26). Try drinking nettle tea, and take a tincture or capsules of devil's claw; ask your herbalist for dosages.

HOT JOINT PROBLEMS

The joints are red and inflamed, particularly during hot and humid weather. For this type of problem, follow a more cooling and yin-enhancing diet (see page 26). Most fruits are helpful, particularly cherries, melon, pawpaw, pears, apples and quinces; also dandelion: either the leaves, added to salads or made into tea; or the roots, in the form of dandelion coffee. If you eat fish, take green lip mussel supplements and cod liver oil. You can apply to the joints a massage oil made with essential oils of mint and lavender. Sometimes a poultice can help the painful joint; try cabbage leaves (see page 94) or clay. Buy the clay from your local chemist or healthfood shop and follow the directions given.

FRACTURES

Follow a wholesome diet which is in harmony with your energy type, because this will build up your vitality and thus help the healing process. Twice a day, between meals, have a tea made from the leaf or root of comfrey; or take tincture of comfrey. Gently massage any area not covered by a plaster cast or bandage with essential oils of cyprus, lavender and sage.

GOUT

Gout is caused by an accumulation of uric acid crystals in a joint, resulting in a red, hot, inflamed condition. It is important to cleanse and cool the liver and kidneys. First of all, particularly during an attack, avoid the following: cheese, red meats, including pork and meat extracts; sardines, mussels, whitebait, herrings, mackerel, anchovies and fish roe; coffee, chocolate, alcohol, sugar and foods which contain it. Follow the advice given for OEDEMA (page 227) to flush out and cleanse the kidneys, and also for OVERHEATED LIVER (page 212). Drink cornsilk tea.

OSTEOPOROSIS (BRITTLE BONES)

This is a condition in which the bones become progressively thinner and more brittle. It is most common in women who have passed the menopause, although it can affect younger women and men too. Sometimes people are advised to increase their intake of calcium and vitamin D.

Although milk and dairy produce are good sources of calcium they have disadvantages in that they are mucus-forming and, unless low-fat varieties are chosen, they can add too much saturated fat to the diet. In addition, they are high in protein, and increasing the daily protein intake beyond a certain level can be counter-productive because the higher the protein intake, the more calcium the body loses each day. Some experts therefore consider it preferable to get your calcium from nuts, seeds, fruits and vegetables. Broccoli is a particularly rich source, as are fresh and dried figs, sesame seeds, tofu and tahini. Include these foods often in a balanced diet such as the one described on pages 31–8. The herb horsetail, taken as a tincture, can be useful in supplementing calcium levels in the body.

Exercise is also important; walking and deep-breathing in the fresh air; yoga or T'ai Chi (see page 270); and relaxation.

CRAMP

Many people suffer from this painful, muscular contraction which affects mainly the calves and feet. It can indicate a deficiency of magnesium and/or calcium, so try taking supplements of these which you can get at your local healthfood shop. You need to take 300–400 mg of magnesium each day, and 800 mg of calcium.

You can also massage the affected area gently, both during a spasm and at other times, as a preventative measure. Once a day, massage your calves and feet with a massage oil containing essential oils of lavender, geranium and camomile.

In Chinese medicine, cramps are often associated with liver and gall bladder imbalances, so read the section on LIVER AND GALL BLADDER PROBLEMS (page 212) and see if you recognise any of the symptoms. You can also try massaging the acupressure point which relates to this condition (liver 3 on an acupressure chart), found between your big toe and the one next to it.

Cancer

There is much evidence linking cancer with diet, environment, lifestyle and stress, as well as hereditary factors; in some cases the evidence is overwhelming but in others it is more tenuous. After many years of research it is now generally accepted that smoking is a contributive factor in lung and mouth cancers as well as other illnesses such as heart disease. But there are many other things, such as chemicals, fumes, dust, radiation and pollution, which may also trigger cancerous growths. Some of these are acknowledged as contributive factors, while others are still disputed; some are man-made, while others (like the ultra-violet rays in sunlight) are natural. Bearing in mind the many colourings, flavourings, additives and preservatives which are added to foods and drinks, as well as the various chemical fertilisers, pesticides and hormones which may be used during the production process, we consider it wise to be cautious and to choose foods which have been produced in as natural a way as possible.

Research among ethnic groups whose diets mainly used to consist of wholegrains, vegetables and pulses showed a very small occurrence of cancer. When these people changed to a low-fibre, high-fat Western-type diet, the incidence of cancerous growths multiplied. A particularly striking example is the Hunza tribe in northern Pakistan, a race of people who lived totally apart from modern civilisation on a simple diet similar to the one described in this book. They were well known for their longevity and were mostly free from serious illnesses. However, modern civilisation finally succeeded in swamping them with food such as ice-creams, colas and hamburgers. Their average lifespan is now greatly reduced and they are dying of the same diseases as us.

So, in our approach to cancer, we have to look at two main aspects: the external causes like chemicals, pollution and lifestyle; and the internal causes of energy imbalances.

On pages 31–8 you will find advice on eating a balanced, healthy diet. Make sure that you completely eliminate sugars, refined grains, mucus-producing foods and all food containing additives. This is a very important step in the prevention and treatment of cancer. Some people might also choose to fast for a few days (see page 40). Various schools of thought sometimes advocate very drastic diets like eating purely raw vegetables and fruits for months, or only boiled rice and vegetables. These sparse regimes can occasionally be very effective, but they can also further exhaust an already weak and depleted body. If you follow a wider but well-balanced cleansing diet you can still achieve good results while keeping your energy level up.

Once you have started following a balanced diet, you need to do a systematic self-diagnosis, as described on page 30, in order to identify your particular energy imbalance and adapt your diet accordingly.

Many patients have found laetrile, or vitamin B17, beneficial, although after brief laboratory tests in the USA B17 supplements were banned by the authorities because they were found to contain cyanide. It is interesting to note, however, that natural sources of B17 (that is, most fruit kernels) also contain cyanide, but the amount is far too low to be harmful and certainly far less toxic than the drugs normally used to treat cancer. Furthermore, tests have shown that the cyanide in kernels is selective, only affecting the cancer cells.

Some of the foods which contain vitamin B17 are shown below. The seeds can be mixed with almonds or cashew nuts and ground up. Take 1 tablespoon of the mixture, sprinkled over your food, twice a day. Do not eat too much B17 rich food if you are also taking laetrile supplements.

FOODS WHICH CONTAIN VITAMIN B17

alfalfa	guavas	Fruit seeds:
almonds	lentils	apple
beet tops	millet	linseed
blackberries	mung beans	apricot
blackcurrants	peas	peach
blackeye beans	raspberries	prune
buckwheat	redcurrants	nectarine
cashew nuts	spinach	
cassava	strawberries	
chickpeas	sweet potatoes	
cranberries	watercress	
gooseberries	yams	

Your natural practitioner might want to prescribe various herbs according to where the growth is, but a good overall herbal combination is: huang chi, red clover, pellitory of the wall, chaparral and figwort. Mix together in equal parts, then boil 1½ tablespoons in 1 litre/1¾ pints water for 5 minutes. Leave to infuse for 15 minutes, then take the mixture over 24 hours. If you are taking this as a tincture, mix the tinctures together, then put 1 tablespoon in 1 litre/1¾ pints water and drink this over 24 hours. In either case, take the mixture at least an hour before or after main meals.

Two Eastern mushrooms have been used throughout the centuries to combat tumours; these are reishi and shiitake. Both are now available in capsule form in many healthfood shops. Dried shiitake can be bought from Chinese shops, and fresh shiitake are sometimes available in supermarkets. Have 50–100 g/2–4 oz fresh or dried shiitake two or three times a week, soaked if dried, then sautéed with a little onion or cooked with other vegetables (see the recipe for SHIITAKE MUSHROOMS WITH SOY SAUCE AND SESAME SEEDS, page 132).

Many studies, particularly in Germany, have also shown beetroot juice to be very effective against cancer. Drink 600 ml/1 pint each day, either during or between meals. You can either buy raw beetroot and juice it yourself, or buy it ready-made in healthfood shops. If you find the taste unbearable, start with half a glass of beetroot juice mixed with another fruit or vegetable juice.

Recently research has been carried out on the effect of beta-carotene foods on cancer and the results are very promising. Foods which are rich in beta-carotene are the dark green and yellow-orange fruits and vegetables: broccoli, spinach, lettuce, watercress, endive, cucumber, carrots, pumpkin, tomatoes, apricots, plums, peaches, cantaloupe melon, mangoes and bananas.

If the tumour is visible under the skin you can apply a poultice to it for a few hours every day. Make this, if possible, with violets and their leaves. If these are not available, you can use cabbage leaves. Soak the flowers and/or leaves for a few minutes, then squeeze a handful of them, adding 2 drops each of essential oils of frankincense, lavender and juniper. Spread a piece of muslin or gauze over the skin, then apply the leaf mixture and cover with another piece of cloth and a bandage. Change every couple of hours.

Finally, we would emphasise the importance of creative visualisation, meditation and gentle exercise (see the chapter on 'Helping the Healing Process', pages 263–73).

Heart and Circulatory System

The heart is an extremely busy organ, pumping large volumes of blood round the body throughout our lives. However, most of us do not do all we can to help this powerful organ to work smoothly. The heart works best in a fit body, where the arteries and other blood vessels are clean and clear of obstructions, and the whole body is supplied with sufficient nutrients. For this to happen, it is most important that the diet only includes moderate quantities of fats and sugars; that the body is exercised regularly but not too strenuously; and that there are no undue stresses. Smoking and alcohol both tax the heart, as do tension and overwork; and both a sedentary lifestyle and over-vigorous exercise can also be detrimental. So it's not surprising that so many people suffer from heart and circulatory problems, all too often leading to premature death or severe illness.

Hardening of the arteries, or ATHEROSCLEROSIS, is largely due to fatty deposits, mainly cholesterol, in their lining. This can cause many further complications like ANEURYSMS (abnormal enlargement of blood vessels); bleeding, ANGINA and THROMBOSIS. Keeping the arteries free from such deposits is vital to a healthy cardio-vascular system. This means following the ANTI-CHOLESTEROL DIET (page 39). Rosehip, hibiscus, cornsilk, fennel and buckwheat teas also help the circulatory system, as does a tea made from dandelion leaves, or the root taken as a coffee substitute. Lecithin supplements, borage seed and/or evening primrose oils are also recommended. Ask your natural practitioner or healthfood shop for products and dosages.

CORONARY ARTERY DISEASE, HEART DISEASE AND ANGINA

If you suspect that you have any of these conditions, you should of course seek prompt medical attention. Dietary and herbal remedies can then be of great benefit in long-term recovery and prevention. As these conditions are mainly due to cholesterol and fatty deposits in the arteries supplying the heart, you should follow the advice given above, to reduce cholesterol and help the circulation. Try drinking, two or three times a week, a weak tea made from equal parts of hawthorn berries and flowers. A few drops of any of the following oils, added to your bath, can also be helpful: lavender, jasmine, geranium and ylang ylang.

HYPERTENSION (HIGH BLOOD PRESSURE)

All the general advice given at the beginning of this section on the heart will greatly benefit high blood pressure conditions. You should also read the advice given under OEDEMA (page 227). Poor kidney function can contribute to high blood pressure, so it is often helpful to have diuretic foods and remedies, thus encouraging the body to get rid of fluid through urination.

Reduction of stress and gentle exercise are also important, and in a number of experiments meditation (see page 271) has been shown to be very helpful in reducing blood pressure. See also TENSION AND STRESS (page 252).

It is helpful to drink teas such as lemon verbena, camomile and orange flower which have a calming effect, particularly if you drink them in the evening. A tea or tincture made with equal parts of hawthorn berries and flowers is good, taken once or twice a day. Onion and garlic, either raw or cooked, are also helpful in the diet.

High blood pressure is very common during pregnancy, especially in the late stages when the body and heart have to cope with a great deal of extra pressure. This condition can be aggravated because pregnant women feel the need to eat more than usual, and turn to refined flour products, sugar and salty convenience foods. The simplest and safest treatment is to eat a balanced wholesome diet as described on pages 31–8. Try to reduce your salt intake as much as possible. Relaxation techniques (see page 271) are also very helpful in pregnancy.

HYPOTENSION (LOW BLOOD PRESSURE)

Slightly lower pressure than normal is not seen as a condition to be worried about; on the contrary some doctors consider it to be a good sign. Excessively low pressure is usually the result of some other health problem, either acute or chronic. For more information on this, see WEAK YANG and WEAK YIN OF THE HEART (page 246).

CIRCULATORY PROBLEMS

VARICOSE VEINS, PHLEBITIS (INFLAMMATION OF THE VEIN WALLS), BROKEN CAPILLARIES, RAYNAUD'S DISEASE (COLD HAND COMPLAINT) and CHILBLAINS are all conditions concerned with the circulation. In order to improve this, the veins and arteries need to be clean and free from deposits; so read and follow the general advice on diet given at the beginning of this section on the heart.

Buckwheat is especially recommended in grain form, and rye is also good; buckwheat leaf tea should be drunk daily by people with circulation problems. Vitamin C supplements are beneficial, as are riboflavonoids (once known as vitamin P and found in the skins of citrus fruit), now available in tablet form. Rutin, a substance which is present naturally in buckwheat and rye, is also helpful; ask your natural practitioner or healthfood shop for products and dosages.

If your circulatory problem is of an inflammatory nature, such as PHLEBITIS, and is made worse by heat and hot weather, you need a more cooling treatment. Follow the diet described at the beginning of this section on the heart, adding a good quantity of salads and fruits, particularly wild berries. Drink buckwheat, rosehip and hibiscus tea frequently. Make up a massage oil using essential oils of lavender and cypress, and apply daily, or three to four times a week, near, but not on top of, the swollen or painful area. Do not massage, as this could exacerbate the condition.

Follow the same advice for BROKEN CAPILLARIES. A tea made with the leaves of either bilberries or strawberries can be helpful.

Do not apply the oil over the leg if there has been a recent swelling or inflammation; wait at least 2 weeks. Instead, follow the diet described at the beginning of this section on the heart and drink once a day, for at least a month, a tea made with equal parts of lime flowers and melilot.

CHILBLAINS are a reaction to excessive coldness affecting the circulation. They can therefore be helped by the application of oils which warm and stimulate the blood. A good combination is equal parts of essential oils of ginger and rosemary added to massage oil in the usual way.

WEAK YANG OF THE HEART

This energy imbalance, or the one which follows, can often be at the root of the problem. Weak yang of the heart could be accompanied by palpitations, pallor, undue sweating on exertion, and sensitivity to cold and fatigue. Read the general advice on diet at the beginning of this section on the heart, and incorporate the dietary suggestions given under TOO LITTLE YANG (page 26).

WEAK YIN OF THE HEART

With this condition there could be palpitations, night sweats, and hot feet and hands, particularly at night. The face may be either red or pale with red cheekbones; and there is likely to be anger alternating with anxiety and fear. Read the general advice on diet at the beginning of this section on the heart, and incorporate the dietary suggestions given under TOO LITTLE YIN (page 26).

Immune System

During the last 15 years or so, diseases such as AIDS and ME have increasingly focused our attention on the importance of the immune system – the organs, cells and antibodies with which the body fights off infections and parasites. The white blood cells (which fight off infective germs) are a major component of the immune system. They are helped in this task by the workings of the skin, respiration, the intestinal flora (the natural bacteria in the gut) and by a harmonious body metabolism. Western and Indian naturopaths place great emphasis on a healthy bowel, while the Chinese consider the lungs to be the site of our defensive energy. So it is not just a question of taking some tablets to increase our immune cell count, but of balancing and strengthening the whole of our systems.

Here are some pointers:

- Many vitamins and minerals have been recommended but there is a general consensus that A, C, E, zinc and selenium are vital for a healthy immune system.
- A shower starting with warm water and ending with a gradual cooling is advised. Also, while having the shower, rub your skin with a hard sponge till you create a warm reddening. This greatly strengthens the skin and the lungs and improves the circulation, as long as the cool shower at the end lasts only a couple of minutes.
- Bowel flora enhancers, like acidopholus, lactobacillus and the juice of aloe vera, are also recommended.
- Follow the advice on pages 31–8 for a generally balanced diet and then look under the relevant chapter to alleviate any condition you might suffer from. Remember that your defences depend mainly on a balanced and vital metabolism.
- The following herbal combination is also useful: 2 parts of huang chi and 1 part each of plantain, borage and echinacea. See page 43 for instructions on preparing tinctures.
- Emotional conflicts and physical tension can weaken our defences; these problems can be relieved by meditation, relaxation techniques and counselling. Regular mild and gentle exercise like walking, swimming, yoga or T'ai Chi should be carried out at least three times a week. Breathing techniques like those used in yoga, even if performed for only 10 minutes a day, are most beneficial. See the chapter on 'Helping the Healing Process' (pages 263–73) and also TENSION AND STRESS (page 252).
- If you live in a city your lungs and blood have to work with polluted air, so try to get fresh air in the countryside, or by the sea, as often as possible. Deep and gentle breathing in clean air will help cleanse your body and strengthen your defences.

ALLERGIES

Rashes, sneezing and streaming eyes are just three of the ways in which the body can show signs of an allergy, and there are many substances, or allergens, which can trigger such reactions. Some of these, such as house dust or certain scents and fumes, are inhaled. For these allergies, which in natural medicine are seen as weaknesses of the immune and respiratory systems, follow the advice given at the beginning of this section on the immune system and under **The Respiratory System** (page 219).

When the allergen is a food or drink, it may be something that is easy to identify, like chocolate, coffee or alcohol. But it is not always so simple to find the culprit. There are many advertisements for methods which purport to do this, but it is difficult to say whether many of them do objectively work or whether they are more dependent on the individual interpretation of the practitioner. Probably the best method is to follow an elimination diet where a particular food is eliminated for a few days and the progress of the condition is followed. If the condition improves while that item is omitted from the diet, and worsens when it is included, then we can clearly say that it is an allergen.

Isolating the allergen, or allergens, is only a part of the therapeutic process; the other part consists of improving the digestive system generally. Read the section on **The Digestive System** (pages 207–18) and follow the advice given. Look also at the section on **The Basic Conditions** (pages 25–30) to find the appropriate diet for your energy type. Some people find that quite soon after they start eating in a healthy, balanced way, allergy problems improve or disappear.

At a mental level, you might find it helpful to examine your life and consider who, or what aspect of it, you are allergic to; whether you are giving away your own power, and if so, how and why. As you find your own strength and inner peace, the allergies may improve, too.

ACQUIRED IMMUNODEFICIENCY SYNDROME (AIDS)

Because so many strong emotions are associated with this condition, it is most valuable to deal with these clearly and honestly, so freeing yourself from the negative aspects of fear.

Read the advice given at the beginning of this section on the immune system. These general points are particularly important for this condition. Then treat your other symptoms individually. For instance, if you have a problem with your lungs, look for your symptoms under **The Respiratory System**, and so on. Read, too, the section on **The Basic Conditions** (pages 25–30).

Because there is a wide variety of symptoms, a diet to help one symptom could aggravate another. For instance, if you eat a lot of cooling and moist foods like fruit and salads, to help weak yin energy which is giving night sweats, you might aggravate a condition like diarrhoea. Therefore it is advisable to follow the ANTI-INFLAMMATION DIET on page 38 and then use the various oils and herbs advised to boost your immunity and treat single conditions like diarrhoea and candidiasis.

MYALGIC ENCEPHALOMYELITIS (ME)

This condition is also known as Post-Viral Syndrome and, in the USA, as Chronic Fatigue Syndrome. It is thought that it may be the result of an initial infection from an influenza virus which goes more deeply into the system, sapping its vitality and leaving the body in a state of near total exhaustion. Doing even simple tasks may bring signs of stress. There is a Catch 22 situation here, for it is necessary to raise the energy level in the body but at the same time the measures which will help this may also create reactions. So it is a question of proceeding slowly but also making sure that progress is made.

Success breeds success, and it is important to take many simple steps towards recovery while at the same time not rushing too fast and collapsing by overdoing things.

If symptoms of colds and fevers persist, follow the advice under COLDS AND FLU (page 219), and make sure you do not come into contact with people carrying viral infections. Also look under **The Basic Conditions** (pages 25–30) to see what sort of constitutional problem you might be having and how to improve it; and read the advice given at the beginning of this section on the immune system, to avoid repeated infections.

In addition to exhaustion, some patients suffer from respiratory or digestive symptoms. In these cases, follow the advice given under **The Respiratory System** (page 219) or **The Digestive System** (page 207) as well. Sometimes the digestion is so greatly affected that patients become strongly allergic to most food; in this case, follow the advice given under ALLERGIES (page 248). If your stomach is so upset that the normal herbal dosages are too strong to take, start with as low a dosage as the body can cope with, and increase it very gradually. Once these respiratory or digestive problems are resolved, keep on following the advice given at the beginning of this section on the immune system. See also the chapter on 'Helping the Healing Process' (pages 263–73).

THYROID DISFUNCTIONS

Thyroid disfunctions are quite common, especially amongst people over 35 years old. If you have any of the symptoms described, it might be worth having a blood test for thyroid functionality. The thyroid abnormalities described do require medical attention, but a wholefood diet and natural treatment could help stop the condition progressing further and also possibly reduce the need for medication.

HYPERTHYROIDISM produces a state of hyperactivity, tension, heat in the system, insomnia and palpitations. Look at the sections on OVERHEATED LIVER (page 212) and WEAK YIN OF THE HEART (page 246). The dietary advice given under these two conditions could definitely be helpful. Stimulants like coffee and alcohol are best eliminated from the diet or greatly reduced; and you are also advised not to take natural stimulants such as guarana or ginseng.

Twice a day, in the morning and evening, take 15 drops of tincture of bugleweed in half a glass of water at least an hour before or after meals.

Before going to bed have a cup of tea made of the following mixture: camomile, hawthorn tops, orange flowers and passiflora. See pages 42–3 for details of making teas.

Relaxation techniques and meditation (see page 271) are very important. It is possible to improve the condition by relaxing from within the mind and body.

In your bath you can use any of the relaxing essential oils like geranium, lavender, camomile, orange flowers or orange peel.

In traditional Chinese medicine HYPOTHYROIDISM is viewed as a deficiency of energy. Look at the section on **The Basic Conditions** (pages 25–30) to see whether you suffer more from lack of yin, yang or blood, and improve your diet, and exercise, accordingly.

Seaweeds are rich in natural iodine, so it is good to include them often in your diet if you suffer from HYPOTHYROIDISM, but be aware too that seaweeds are very cooling and prolonged use can cause a lack of vitality. You can take up to four kelp tablets a day, preferably two at lunch and two at dinner.

Lymphatic System

The lymphatic system is a network of interconnecting channels throughout the body; in between the channels are small bean-shaped nodules called lymph nodes which are mainly composed of lymphocytes, a type of white blood cell. The function of the lymph system is to fight infection in the body; it plays an important part in cleansing our bodies and boosting immunity. When there is a wound, the lymph nodes nearby become active, swollen and tender as the lymphocytes multiply to fight the infection. The swelling subsides once the infection has disappeared or the wound has healed.

People with weak constitutions or immunity might suffer from a sluggish lymphatic system. They are inclined to have frequent, repeated colds, weak digestion and low vitality, and the lymph nodes tend to get swollen and tender. If they eat a wholesome diet, in harmony with their constitution, the lymphatic system will respond. See also the advice given at the beginning of the section on **The Immune System** (page 246).

As well as a balanced diet, the following foods are quite useful for cleansing the lymphatic system: watercress, dandelion, nettle, seaweeds, celery, wild chicory, artichoke, cabbage, onions, leeks, lemons, limes, peaches, plums, melon, watermelon and wild berries. You can also have a tea made with echinacea and cornsilk. See pages 42–3 for how to make teas. Take this twice a day, a couple of hours before or after meals.

A massage, once or twice a month, along the lymph network, starting from the feet, and ending below the clavicle, or collar bone is also recommended. Many people who practise massage know this pathway; you could have regular treatments or you could learn how to do the massage and do it yourself with some essential oils and the help of a partner. The best massage oil to prepare for this is a combination of equal parts of essential oils of lavender, geranium and juniper. However, this massage must not be used in the case of cancer because it could encourage metastasis, or the spread of the malignancy through the body.

Remember that the lymphatic system has no pumping mechanism; it relies for its flow on the strength of the surrounding muscles, so mild but regular exercise is very important for its health.

Nervous System

TENSION AND STRESS

Of all the conditions of sickness and ill-health it is those which affect our nerves and emotions in which we can see most clearly the very strong links between our mind, our emotional nature and our physical body.

Modern life has greatly increased the stress experienced by most of us, both because of the speed at which we work and play, and also because of the ways in which we pollute our environment. The pollutants in the air we breathe, the water we drink and the food we eat affect our bodies and take away some of the energy and vitality we need to deal with life.

So it is very important to check that you are doing everything you can to help yourself. Rest; clean, wholesome food and drink; exercise in the fresh air; harmony; peace of mind: all these will help you to be healthy, as will energy-raising activities such as yoga and T'ai Chi, and meditation and relaxation techniques (see the chapter on 'Helping the Healing Process', pages 263–73).

There are some physical conditions which may linger undiagnosed and make us unhappy. These include premenstrual tension, thyroid disfunction and atherosclerosis. So if you are feeling unduly unhappy, depressed, or tense, it is worth checking to see if you are suffering from a physical ailment.

According to Chinese medicine, all the basic energy imbalances described on pages 25–30 can create emotional conflicts, and by harmonising the energy, the emotional state can be improved. It is impossible to illustrate all the possible connections between energy imbalances and emotions in a few pages, but here are a few brief pointers:

- WEAK YANG ENERGY can create a state of coldness and weakness in the system. There is lack of assertion, self-confidence and will-power; apathy and lack of sexual drive. The symptoms tend to get worse in the winter. See TOO LITTLE YANG (page 26), WEAK YANG OF THE KIDNEYS (page 224), and WEAK YANG OF THE HEART (page 246).
- EXCESSIVE HEAT can give a feeling of being quite hot. The face is red; sometimes the eyes are bloodshot. There may be 'bursting'-type headaches. This condition creates rather an aggressive, manic and restless type of personality which is quick to anger. See TOO MUCH YANG AND HEAT (page 25), HOT DIGESTION (page 208) and OVERHEATED LIVER (page 212).

- STAGNANT ENERGY is a very common condition which relates to accumulated emotion blocking the system. The person tends to be tense, restless and easily frustrated. There is often swelling and flatulence in the abdomen. See STAGNANT ENERGY IN THE DIGESTION (page 208) and STAGNANT ENERGY IN THE LIVER (page 213).
- WEAK YIN ENERGY can create dryness, a sensation of heat in the afternoons, night sweats and anxiety, fear, irritation and listlessness. See TOO LITTLE YIN (page 26), WEAK YIN OF THE KIDNEYS (page 225) and WEAK YIN OF THE HEART (page 246).
- WEAK BLOOD gives pallor, brittle nails and hair. The person often feels tired and dizzy. The condition is common amongst women and they could feel more tired during and just after a period. The person lacks self-confidence and is quite vulnerable. See EMPTY OR WEAK BLOOD (page 30).

If you cannot identify with any of these types, do not worry. If you follow the general guidance given in this section and also that given in the section on eating a balanced diet (pages 31–8), you will be able to improve the workings of your nervous system and soothe your emotions. The following foods and remedies are particularly good for the nervous system, but need to be used in conjunction with a balanced diet and a healthy way of life which includes walking often in the open air; mild exercises and meditation (see page 271).

Some of the most valuable foods for the nervous system are the wholegrains because of their high vitamin B content. Oats and wheatgerm are especially good. Lecithin is valuable and can be taken as a supplement, although soya and its derivatives (such as tofu and miso) also contain it, as does soy sauce. However, miso and soy sauce should be taken in moderation because of their high salt content. Supplements of vitamin B complex and vitamin E can also be helpful.

Recommended vegetables include carrots, celery, courgettes, lettuce and pumpkin; fruits, such as apricots, peaches, melon, pawpaw, quinces, figs, avocados, mandarins and tangerines; seeds and nuts are a concentrated source of helpful nutrients, especially almonds, sesame seeds and sunflower seeds. Spices which are particularly valuable are aniseed, camomile, lemon verbena, mint, rose petals, orange peel and flowers, marjoram, rosemary, sage and basil; and the following essential oils: lavender, geranium, rose, orange flowers (sometimes called neroli), orange peel and camomile. Add these to your bath; sprinkle them on a handkerchief or pillow; or add them to massage oil and rub them over your skin.

INSOMNIA

Read the above section carefully because insomnia often indicates an underlying cause or deeper imbalance which needs to be dealt with. However, you should also make sure that the insomnia is actually a problem and is not simply a sign that you do not need much sleep. Some people really can do with far less sleep than others, particularly if they are able to recharge their energy through meditation.

If your energy is too tense then do follow the advice given at the beginning of this section on the nervous system. Relaxation and meditation (see page 271) will be particularly helpful in calming your energy. Make sure that you do not aggravate the condition by eating too late in the evening or too unwisely. Teas made from camomile, lemon verbena or orange flowers taken before going to bed can be very helpful. Alternatively, a combination of passiflora and skullcap would be a little stronger.

MULTIPLE SCLEROSIS (MS)

This condition can be greatly helped by a wholefood diet, particularly when this is started in the early stages of the disease. Read carefully the section on **The Basic Conditions** (pages 31–8) and adopt a wholesome diet in accordance with your own energy type. Read also the general guidance on foods which help the nervous system (page 253). Exercises like swimming and walking, to strengthen the muscular, cardio-vascular and respiratory systems, are advised, and also those which balance and invigorate the nervous system, such as yoga and T'ai Chi (see page 270). Oil of evening primrose can be extremely helpful and, as part of an overall healthy lifestyle, can help to stabilise the condition.

MEMORY WEAKENING

Follow the advice given at the beginning of this section on the nervous system; this will greatly help your memory and brain power. It is important to encourage a good flow of blood to the head, so see also **The Heart and Circulatory System** (pages 243–6). Any of the following herbs, taken as a mild tea, can be helpful: sage, rosemary, marjoram or basil. Use a quarter of a teaspoonful of the dried herb to a cup of freshly boiled water and infuse for 5 minutes. These herbs can also be used in the form of essential oils, added to a carrier oil and massaged over the neck and forehead. It may be beneficial to add 5 drops to your bath.

HYPERACTIVITY

Hyperactivity in children frequently improves dramatically with a change of diet. Ice lollies and sweets made from sugar and dye should be eliminated from the diet, as should all foods containing artificial colouring, white sugar, additives and preservatives; and too many fried foods. These foods, which ruin their teeth, rattle their nerves, upset their digestions and give them allergies, are best replaced by healthy treats: ice lollies made from pure fruit juices (home-made or available from some shops); sugarless carob bars; cakes made with wholewheat flour and honey or real brown sugar; and dried fruits. In general the diet should be based on wholefoods, with plenty of grains, vegetables and fruit, as described on pages 31–8.

These principles not only apply to children, but also to adults with tense, hyperactive nervous systems.

ALZHEIMER'S DISEASE (SENILITY)

If this condition is caught early on, it can be improved by natural medicine. It is important to keep a good flow of blood to the head, so a diet which keeps the arteries elastic and free from deposits is most helpful (see **The Heart and Circulatory System**, page 243). It is helpful, too, to keep the neck relaxed and flexible with massage and gentle exercise because this improves the circulation to the head. Massage the shoulders, neck and forehead with an essential oil dilution of basil and rosemary. Use 6 drops of each in 100 ml/3½ fl oz massage oil.

Some researchers believe that aluminium deposits in the system play a part in the disease. Whilst more studies need to be done on this, it might be wise to avoid cooking, especially acid food, or brewing tea, in aluminium utensils. Some people would go so far as to say that it is best to avoid boiling water in aluminium kettles, too.

Very good results have been obtained with a supplement made from

255

the leaves of the ginkgo biloba tree and many practitioners are now recommending this for sufferers from Alzheimer's disease.

NEURITIS (NEURALGIA)

Unless the pain comes from a trauma or blow, or a mechanical problem in the back like sciatica, nerve inflammation is generally considered to be a condition of excessive heat. Whatever the cause, this condition can be helped by the ANTI-INFLAMMATION diet (page 38). If you think you have a condition of excessive heat in any of your organs, follow the advice given under TOO MUCH YANG AND HEAT (page 25). You can add to this regime a tea made from St John's wort which should be taken twice a day, at least an hour before or after meals. Alternatively, you can take this as a tincture, adding the drops to water.

An ointment or massage oil made with essential oils of lavender and camomile is soothing. Apply some oil or ointment to the painful area night and morning.

ANOREXIA NERVOSA

This is quite a complex psycho-physical condition which requires a great deal of caring both by those close to the sufferer and by practitioners. Often anorexia can alternate with BULIMIA NERVOSA, a condition in which the person makes themselves sick or takes laxatives after an eating binge. The main danger in anorexia nervosa is that the person could suffer from severe malnutrition, with serious health complications. For this reason, and because, when they do accept food, it is usually in small amounts, make sure that it is very nourishing.

Avoid stodgy foods such as white pasta and cakes; think in terms of vegetable juices, preferably fresh, if you have a juicer, with some wheatgerm sprinkled into them. Or fizzy vitamins could be added to the juices; vitamins C, E and A, and zinc, are considered important for this condition. You can also try making a soup with various mixed vegetables, then, 5 minutes before it is ready, add some oats and oat bran; at the end, add wheatgerm and a little yeast. Try giving them salads, beanburgers, a little steamed fish, if they eat this, a little hummus, or some omelette sprinkled with GOMASIO or sesame seed salt (see page 172).

In both anorexia and bulimia there is usually a great deal of anger and depression. These are emotions which in Chinese medicine denote congestion in the liver and a weakness in the pancreas. Read the advice under LIVER AND GALL BLADDER PROBLEMS (page 212). Of course techniques to soothe the mind and free the emotions are most important; these would include counselling, yoga, T'ai Chi, relaxation, visualisation, meditation and massage (see the chapter on 'Helping the Healing Process', pages 263–73). Try to encourage the patient not to lock themselves up inside the house; country walks and mild exercise in the fresh air are helpful.

OBESITY

It feels miserable to be overweight, as well as putting unnecessary stress on all the systems of the body. Losing weight is not particularly easy because it means breaking the habits which have led to the weight gain and adapting to a new way of eating. This can however be tremendously rewarding, for not only will you lose weight steadily and look better and better, but, if you choose a healthy, balanced diet, you will also begin to feel better and you will develop a way of eating which will enable you to remain slim and healthy.

Nervous and emotional factors are often at the root of weight problems, and it may be helpful to look at these. Try not to resist the weight, but to love and accept yourself as you are at each stage of your diet. This will help you to lose weight, as will being aware of your feelings, whether these are anger, guilt, resentment, fear, a sense of worthlessness, or whatever. Accepting the feelings, and realising that you have every right to feel them, takes the power out of them. It may not make them go away, but it defuses them, and brings a sense of peace and wellbeing. The Bach flower remedies (see page 269) can be helpful for dealing with the moods, emotions and mental states which can wreck a diet; see also Rose Elliot's *Vegetarian Slimming* (under Further Reading) for more about using these.

Although it can be a good idea to start a long-term weight loss programme with a few days of controlled FASTING (see page 40), short-term starvation diets are not helpful because they give a feeling of deprivation leading to bingeing, with consequent guilt, followed by more deprivation and so on. What is needed is a balanced diet which restores harmony and gives adequate nourishment, along with gentle yet regular weight loss.

It is best to follow a diet which is both in harmony with your energy type (see **The Basic Conditions**, pages 25–30) and low in mucus-forming foods (see the ANTI-MUCUS DIET, page 39). You can have low-fat milk products, but even these are best taken in great moderation. Have a little skimmed milk in your drinks if you must, and low-fat yogurt and cottage cheese in moderation.

Try basing your meals mainly on natural wholegrains, particularly brown rice; or, for a change, baked or boiled potatoes or sweetcorn, or polenta; and porridge made from oatmeal for breakfast. Have small quantities of tofu, cooked beans, peas or lentils, or a tablespoonful of sesame salt or seeds, sunflower or pumpkin seeds, chopped walnuts or grated almonds for protein; or small quantities of fish and chicken if you eat these.

Include in each meal as many vegetables as you fancy, steamed in 1–2 tablespoons boiling stock or stir-fried in 1 teaspoon olive oil. Vegetables which are particularly helpful for weight loss are artichokes, asparagus, celery, chicory, cucumber, dandelion, fennel, leeks, lettuce, onions, seaweeds, spinach, tomatoes and watercress; and for flavouring, bay leaf, fennel seed, horseradish and parsley. Eat fruit in moderation, perhaps one piece a day, as it is quite high in sugar and thus in calories. Particularly good are apples, bilberries, cherries, grapefruit, lemons and limes, peaches, pears, plums and prunes.

You need not restrict your fluid intake as long as it is water or water-based and not sweetened with honey, sugar or artificial sweeteners; fruit juices, too, are best avoided. Rosehip and hibiscus tea are particularly beneficial and can be drunk freely; try also a cup of tea made from fennel seed or bay leaf, and 1–2 cups of dandelion coffee a day.

If you find that your problem is simply eating too much at meals, try taking one of the products such as guar gum, which you can get at healthfood shops, and which swell inside your stomach. These are also a source of natural fibre, so they are good for the intestines, and they inhibit the absorption of fats.

Do all you can to build up your confidence and to make life pleasant and easy for yourself while you are dieting. Spoiling yourself as you would a loved one, giving yourself little non-food treats, such as flowers, scent, a magazine, some fragrant bath oil or a bubble bath, helps to keep up morale. Essential oils can help, too; try lavender, camomile, geranium or bergamot to lift your spirits; frankincense to help you break old habits, or rose, which is very expensive, but wonderfully soothing and cherishing. Use the oils singly or mixed, added to massage oil and rubbed on your body; sprinkled on a cotton handkerchief, or added to your bath.

Headaches and Migraine

Headaches are most often due to excessive accumulated tension and strain, and also a diet which is causing an energy imbalance in the body, especially in the digestive organs. Many people spend their days under pressure, keeping themselves going with coffee and chocolate and then drinking heavily in the evenings in order to unwind. Headaches are their body's way of telling them to calm down and relax, but instead of listening to these warnings they swallow pain-killers and continue in the same way. Of course there can be other more serious underlying causes such as brain tumours and meningitis and these need urgent medical attention. It should also be mentioned that many physical conditions can give pain in the head as a side effect. When the main cause disappears the headaches clear up too.

Here we are dealing with the most likely causes of headaches and migraines which can be helped through self-treatment. Apart from stress, inflammation of the sinuses, premenstrual tension (PMT) and high blood pressure are common causes; arthritis or joint restrictions in the neck can also cause discomfort in the head, especially around the back of the head or the skull. For more about these, see the relevant sections in this book.

In order to get relief from headaches and migraines you will need to make changes in your diet and reduce your stress level. Coffee, chocolate, fried and fatty food and white sugar need to be eliminated; alcohol and red meat should be taken only in moderation and avoided altogether during attacks. It is also worth checking whether any medicinal drugs, hormones or foods you may be taking could be triggering this problem. In our opinion the best way to find out about allergies is an elimination diet where you avoid the suspected item for a few days and monitor your condition to see whether it improves. In addition to this, follow a balanced, health-giving diet, with regular meals, as described on pages 31–8.

Headaches due to stress, over-concentration and eye-strain can be treated by relaxation exercises, disciplines such as T'ai Chi, and yoga, or meditation (see the chapter on 'Helping the Healing Process', pages 263–73). Regular swimming, getting out into the open air frequently, and having a massage or aromatherapy treatment from time to time, can be beneficial too. It's also helpful to practise massaging your own neck and shoulder area; breathe gently and deeply and notice when you are beginning to accumulate tension so that you can release it straight away by relaxing your body and harmonising your breath. Getting a good night's sleep is also important; try drinking a relaxing tea like camomile, lemon verbena, lemon balm or orange flower.

In the past few years we have heard much about the beneficial effects of plants in the chrysanthemum family: in particular, *Chrysanthemum parthenium* or feverfew, widely used in the West; and *Chrysanthemum morifolium* or ju hua, used in China and the Far East, but now available in the West too. Western tradition has maintained that these plants are warming, whilst its Eastern counterpart categorises them as slightly cold. In our experience, they are more neutral in action, which is why they can relieve headaches and migraines in so many people. We suggest that you first try feverfew, and if this does not work, try ju hua. These remedies are helpful for headaches and migraines caused by stress, allergies, tension colds, sinusitis, imbalances in the digestive system and PMT. They must not be used during pregnancy or if there is excessive menstrual bleeding.

Traditional Chinese medicine can give us some very good clues as to how to treat headaches and migraines according to their location and sensation. Pain in the head which feels sore and constricting is mainly due to stagnation of energy caused by stress, tension and irregular eating patterns. If it is around the forehead, it is thought to be due to stagnation of stomach and colon energy. Follow the advice given under INDIGESTION (page 207). This kind of pain on the top and sides of the head is usually due to stagnation of energy in the liver and gall bladder (see LIVER AND GALL BLADDER PROBLEMS, page 212). For both these conditions, the following teas are recommended: orange peel, mandarin peel and mint, for smooth functioning of the liver and stomach; fennel, cardamom and coriander, to encourage the food to move down from the stomach; and aniseed, camomile and lemon verbena which help ease a constricted digestion due to nervous tension.

Pain of a 'bursting' nature is usually due to heat in the system; check to make sure that you haven't got high blood pressure. This type of pain in the forehead is usually due to heat in the stomach or colon (see HOT DIGESTION, page 208). 'Bursting' pain on the sides and top of the head could be due to heat in the liver and gall bladder (see OVERHEATED LIVER AND GALL BLADDER, page 212). As well as following the relevant advice for these conditions, take the chrysanthemum teas described above and also try tea made from speedwell.

Dull pain in the head is due to weak energy, weak blood or anaemia: see EMPTY OR WEAK BLOOD (page 30), TOO LITTLE YANG (page 26) and WEAK YANG OF THE HEART (page 246).

Childhood Diseases

ERUPTIVE DISEASES

This group consists of diseases such as measles, chicken pox, rubella and scarlet fever, in which there is a fever and a rash or skin eruption and you should of course get medical advice.

In Chinese medicine, such diseases are believed to be the result of toxins which accumulate in the baby's body whilst it is in the womb. So the disease itself is regarded as a cleansing process which is triggered by a virus, and a step towards health and well-being. Treatment therefore concentrates on cooling the fever and helping to draw out the skin eruption. The diet should be cooling; CLEAR VEGETABLE BROTH (page 86) or soups, perhaps with added grains, such as oats or barley; cooked rice; BARLEY WATER (page 154); fruit juice in moderation (because it is so high in sugar), perhaps diluted with still or fizzy mineral water.

In the first stage, when there is a fever, tinctures of boneset, catmint and elderflowers, can be given. These will help to reduce the fever. During the eruptive period you can add burdock to the mixture. Once they reach the convalescent stage, give these tinctures, to help build them up: huang chi, borage and plantain, together with some multi-vitamins for children.

MUMPS

In mumps, there is usually swelling of the salivary glands, together with a fever. Again, natural treatment can be given alongside that advised by the doctor; this treatment involves reducing the fever and cleansing the lymphatic system. Follow the dietary suggestions already given for ERUPTIVE DISEASES (see above) and give a mixture of the following tinctures: boneset, elderflowers, catmint and poke root. You can massage the body gently with an essential oil combination of ti tree, lavender and geranium.

WHOOPING COUGH

If whooping cough is caught at the very beginning, before the barking stage has set in, natural remedies can be quite helpful, used in conjunction with normal medical treatment. As with any cough with mucus, dairy produce should be eliminated from the diet, except for the occasional yogurt. Avoid refined grains such as white pasta; white sugar and anything which contains it; fatty foods such as fish and chips, pork and products made from it, see the ANTI-MUCUS DIET (page 39). Give CLEAR VEGETABLE BROTH (page 86) and soups; cooling foods, particularly grains; and fruit such as grapes to nibble. If the child eats animal proteins, they can have a little fish.

The following tinctures can be given, mixed in equal parts: marshmallow, violet leaves, coltsfoot and elecampane. You can massage the chest and back gently with Vick vapour rub or Olbas, or the following essential oils mixed in a carrier oil: eucalyptus, sage and frankincense.

Keep the room vaporised by placing a saucer of water over a radiator; or use an essential oil burner which you can buy quite cheaply. This consists of a cup-like compartment set over a nightlight. The ceramic type are good; choose one which has a good deep cup or you will be forever topping up the water. You can add to the water a few drops of the essential oils suggested above, to scent as well as vaporise the room, and help the healing process. You can also use essential oils of lavender and frankincense to make a massage oil for the chest and back.

If you follow these suggestions, along with any medical advice you may be given, the attack should clear up fairly quickly. If it goes into the dry, barking phase, use the following tinctures: marshmallow, violet leaves, coltsfoot, lobelia and lemon balm. These can be taken in the form of tea if tinctures are not available.

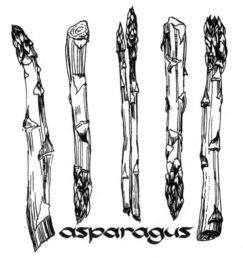

asparagus

5

Helping the Healing Process

Although this book is mainly about treatment with diet, healing the body is inextricably linked with healing other aspects of ourselves. You can certainly help the process by working within as well, looking at the emotional and mental states which may be connected with your illness.

The Body–Mind Balance

In traditional Chinese medicine, major organs in the body are regarded as the physical manifestation of various emotions. Organs which are functioning normally and healthily correspond to a positive emotion or mental attitude such as hopefulness and joy; and when they are diseased, they correspond to the opposite, such as pessimism or sadness.

As explained on page 23, the healing process can begin with either the physical or the emotional aspect of the disease. As the organ becomes well, the negative expression of the emotion associated with it is replaced by the positive one. And the process can work the other way; replacing a negative emotion with its positive equivalent can help to heal the organ associated with it. So healing can start either with the physical body or in the mind and emotions – or in both at the same time.

This approach is very similar to modern holistic healing which diagnoses not only the physical problem but also the emotional and mental state of the person. In her book *You Can Heal Your Life*, Louise L. Hay takes the process even further, linking many illnesses with the thought patterns which may have contributed to them and showing how, by changing the thought, we can change the condition.

The Chinese philosophy linking the emotions with organs of the body evolved over thousands of years and is quite complex, so we can only offer a very simplified introduction here.

The organs are considered in pairs – lungs and large intestine, heart and small intestine, liver and gall bladder, kidney and bladder, stomach and pancreas – and each organ is associated with a particular emotion.

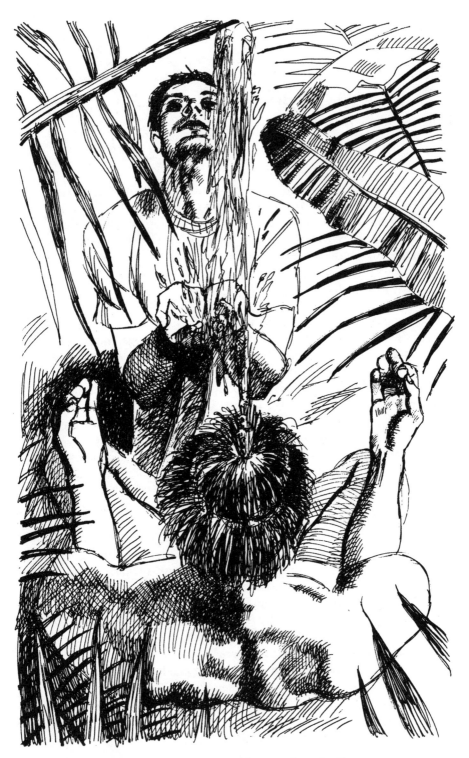

Shiva healing a pilgrim with water from the Ganges

At the end of the description of each pair of organs, you will find a suggested affirmation. An affirmation is a positive statement which, when repeated many times, helps to bring about that condition. You can make up your own affirmation, playing around with different words until they sound right to you. Keep the wording as short as possible, so that you can remember it and quickly bring it to mind. Also, be sure that the affirmation is positive. For instance, instead of saying 'I am not unhappy', you would say 'I am happy'.

You can spend a few minutes a day, perhaps before you go to sleep at night, or after a period of meditation (see page 271), repeating your affirmation. Or you can simply bring it to mind whenever a negative or fearful thought comes to you. Just watch, though, that in doing this you are not refusing to acknowledge a negative feeling or fear which needs to be looked at and worked through before you can let it go. If this is the case, a good counsellor might be able to help you.

There are no 'wrong' emotions, but bottling up feelings because they are too painful to look at creates disharmony in our being. Whilst we are denying, suppressing or repressing feelings we are closing off from part of ourselves; we are not whole. Confronting the negative feelings like anger, guilt and fear – which we all have – takes courage but leads to optimum health.

Learning to feel the feelings but not to be swept away by them or compelled to react to them is a sign of emotional health, as is the capacity to have intimate, fulfilled personal relationships. The realisation that we are responsible for how we feel and that no one can make us angry, hurt, upset, happy or unhappy is both freeing and empowering. As you look at your feelings and communicate them, preferably directly to the person concerned (or in writing or drawing), then let them go, you will feel an increasing sense of inner peace, vitality and well-being in your body.

LUNGS AND LARGE INTESTINE

When the lungs are functioning in a healthy, harmonious way, they perform the essential task of taking new air into the body. At a mental and emotional level this corresponds with our ability to open ourselves to new experiences and possibilities. In order to do that, we need to recycle, eliminate or let go of those things of the past – emotions, beliefs and habits – which are no longer needed.

In the same way, the large intestine, through its function of eliminating waste from the body, creates more space for the lungs to receive new air. Very constipated people find it quite difficult to take a deep breath, and constipation can be helped by deep breathing from the abdomen. We help our lungs to be healthy by having a clean, clear colon. When the lungs are in disharmony, a person tends to feel sad and to slouch. They are in a state of sorrow, feeling that something in the past has crushed them, or that they have been unable to accept a loss or disappointment.

In Chinese medicine, honeysuckle tea is considered to be very good for the lungs; in the BACH FLOWER REMEDIES (see page 269), honeysuckle is the main remedy given to help people let go of memories of the past; and as you walk past a hedge of honeysuckle, the fragrance makes you open your heart and chest.

Affirmations
For the lungs: Take a deep breath, feel the life-force entering your body and say 'I am open to new spaces, dimensions and opportunities in my life.'
For the colon: 'I let go of the past and of past conditioning.'

HEART AND SMALL INTESTINE

The heart is considered to be the site of the spirit, and it relates to how we feel about ourselves. So a person with healthy heart energy has lustre in their eyes and a sense of *joie de vivre*. When there is too little energy in the heart, people lack enthusiasm, they don't like themselves and life seems very dull and sad.

Sometimes there can be excess energy in the heart. Usually this is excess yang energy, which the Chinese call 'over joy'. This is characteristic of people who drive themselves too hard and always want to be on a high, with a hyped-up, 'wired' level of energy – the classic 'work-hard, play-hard' type. This can tax the physical heart a great deal, because we need to go into lower levels of energy in order to relax and allow our body to regenerate itself. Such hyped-up conditions usually show that there is too much heat and yang energy, so look up WEAK YIN OF THE HEART (page 246) for advice on cooling the heart and increasing its yin energy.

Physically, the job of the small intestine is to extract the nutrients from food and then take into the large intestine whatever needs to be eliminated from the system. This coincides with its emotional function, which is discrimination, or the separating of good from bad (it is sometimes known as 'the inner judge'). So when the small intestine is in harmony, we know instinctively what can improve and enhance our life, and this nourishes our spirit, the heart. But when it is in disharmony, we experience confusion about our values, and that dulls the spirit. To improve matters, follow the advice given under INDIGESTION (page 207).

Affirmations

For the heart: 'My own light shines in my heart and I share it with the world' or 'My heart is filled with love and I share it with the world.'
For the small intestine: 'I discriminate with love and I only take what is good for me.'

LIVER AND GALL BLADDER

The liver is like a large furnace which cleanses the system and stores nutrients to be used in various parts of the body. The Chinese believe that the liver stores information which we can use to make plans and programme our life. So if the liver is in harmony, a person can easily make plans and know in which direction they are going.

The gall bladder is supposed to give us the final push needed to put our plans into practice. So when the gall bladder is healthy, we can do what we intend to do. If the liver and gall bladder are not functioning properly, or if our plans keep getting thwarted, we begin to feel very frustrated and angry, we do not know where to go and we cannot fulfil our intentions. Look at the section on LIVER AND GALL BLADDER PROBLEMS (page 212) and try the following affirmations.

Affirmations

For the liver: 'I feel guided and I know my path in life' or 'My inner guidance shows me my path in life.'
For the gall bladder: 'I am able to manifest my plans fully in my life.'

KIDNEY AND BLADDER

The kidneys, situated in the lower back, one on each side of the spine, sustain both our yang and yin energy. The yang of the kidneys is connected with our willpower. It is usually an energy which rises from the base of the spine and moves into the chest. It gives us warmth, confidence and courage, as well as sexual and reproductive power. The yin aspect of the kidneys gives coolness to the body and a strength which comes from inner peace and calmness. A good yin energy enables us to be at peace in a fiery, angry situation. People with weak yin energy are easily upset by such situations.

The balance of yin and yang in the kidneys affects the balance of yin and yang throughout the body. The function of the bladder is rather like that of the gall bladder, in that it helps us to actualise the will of the kidneys, or to bring about in our lives those things which we want to happen.

Affirmations

For the kidneys: 'My will is the expression of my true being and creates harmony.'
To raise the yin of the kidneys: 'I manifest my strength with inner peace.'
For the bladder: 'I manifest my will in the world for the greater good of myself and those around me.'

STOMACH AND SPLEEN/PANCREAS

The ancients used to compare the stomach to a father or provider who went to look for food. Emotionally, the stomach has to do with our capacity for self-esteem, our willingness to receive, to fend for ourselves, and to provide. The spleen and pancreas, which the Chinese always considered together, are linked to the mother, or the one who distributes the food with fairness and sympathy to the children. So the spleen/pancreas show our capacity for sympathy, fairness, clear thought and optimism.

When the stomach is in disharmony, we are unable to fend for ourselves; we are not sure where our place is in the world, and we are not willing to receive help. A classic case of this is the anorexic, who has an unwillingness to receive and does not know where they are. When the pancreas is not functioning well, as people with sugar imbalances know only too well, the ability to concentrate is affected and there is a tendency to depression. Because of this disturbed mental state, the mother-like sympathy for others is often lacking, and there is muddle and confusion.

Affirmations

For the stomach: 'I know my place in the world and all my needs are met.'

For the pancreas/spleen: 'I have sympathy for all life and my thinking is clear.'

STAGNANT BLOOD AND MUCUS

There is one other condition which is not related to any particular organ but has a secondary connection with stagnation of liver energy and a weak pancreas; and that is stagnant blood and mucus which the Chinese believe can create either benign or malignant growths. This often comes about because we feel stuck in a situation in our lives and completely at a loss as to what to do. For this, it is more important than ever to practise the meditation given on page 271. We also need to let go of the past and pray for, or open ourselves to, guidance in our lives – then be ready to see it when it comes! For this condition, the following affirmation can be used.

Affirmation
'I follow my inner being and my energy flows freely.'

BACH FLOWER REMEDIES

Dr Edward Bach discovered this system of healing which consists of remedies made from plants, flowers and trees. There are 38 remedies in all and one composite treatment, RESCUE REMEDY, which is made up from five of the others and is particularly useful for treating shock. These remedies can be extraordinarily effective, either used on their own or alongside other treatments. You can buy the remedies and a simple guide to using them (see Judy Howard's *The Bach Flower Remedies Step by Step* under Further Reading) or you can write to the Edward Bach Centre, Mount Vernon, Sotwell, Wallingford, Oxon. OX10 0PZ.

When there is a clear link between a disease and an emotional or mental state, the Bach Flower Remedies can be a particularly helpful part of the treatment. In fact they work well for all sorts of illnesses and ailments. However, they are always prescribed for the mental or emotional state of the person, rather than their physical symptoms.

Treatment Through Exercise

Exercising the body can help to move blocked energy and get the life force flowing. The important thing is to find a system of exercise which feels right for you, whether it is bioenergetics, T'ai Chi Ch'uan, yoga or some other activity. Follow your instinct when making your choice. Then start your exercise gently, perhaps just five minutes a day, gradually increasing the time as you enjoy it more and more – and feel the benefit.

BIOENERGETICS

Bioenergetics was developed by Dr Alexander Lowen following the work of Wilhelm Reich. It is based on the principle that if energy is blocked in its expression, usually as a result of emotional or mental traumas, it becomes trapped in the body and is not then available to the person to use in his or her life. This energy can, however, be released by exercising in special ways, and this is often also accompanied by release of the emotions which originally caused the blocks. Bioenergetics is very freeing, simple to do, and can sometimes help to cure long-standing ailments. For more information on bioenergetics, see the books by Alexander Lowen under Further Reading.

T'AI CHI CH'UAN

T'ai Chi is a form of martial art in which the exercises and movements are designed to raise the energy and strengthen the body, to sharpen the mind, and also to help the practitioner become aware of his or her deeper spiritual nature. Much attention is paid to the breathing during the movements, and this seems to contribute to the resulting feeling of well-being and power. As with all these activities the more you practise the greater the benefits you will receive. For more information on T'ai Chi, see the books by Da Liu and Chee Soo under Further Reading.

YOGA

At first glance, yoga may appear to be simply a series of physical postures – some sitting, some standing, some lying, some inverted – which stretch, relax and strengthen the body. However, it can also produce a sense of great peace and well-being, as well as stimulating vital glands and organs in the body. For more information on yoga, see the books by Jenny Beeken, Sophy Hoare and B. K. S. Iyengar under Further Reading.

Relaxation, Meditation and Visualisation

In a diseased patient there is mental and emotional tension, constricted breathing, and a tense body. If we can release these tensions the energy can flow, and as it flows it brings healing. Tension can be helped by exercise, as described above, and also by relaxation and meditation. In China today there are hospitals in which cancer patients have been helped by a combination of meditation and Chi Gong (a system of meditative exercises done with a calm mind and a steady breath in which the energy is encouraged to flow to all parts of the body).

A daily or twice-daily period of relaxation and meditation can certainly be a very helpful part of the healing process; and whether or not you believe that these can actually make you better, there is plenty of evidence to suggest that they can improve the quality of your life. The technique which we describe here for relaxation, meditation and visualisation is one which is simple but effective. There are of course many different ways of meditating, and if you would like to know more about these do refer to some of the books suggested under Further Reading. A particularly helpful one is *How to Meditate – A Guide to Self-Discovery* by Laurence LeShan.

It's easiest to relax when you are lying down on your back, or in a position that is comfortable for you, tucked up in a blanket or cover, so that you are quite warm. Now let every part of your body flop, so that it feels really heavy, as though it is going to sink through the floor. You can think of each part of your body in turn, starting with your toes and working right up to your scalp (not forgetting your face, jaw and tongue, which can be very tense), gently telling them to relax and let go of all tension. Or you can tense and then relax each part of your body, again starting with your toes.

By the end of this process you may well have slipped off into a peaceful sleep. If not, this is a time when you can gently concentrate on your breathing, or enjoy a period of visualisation, or say any affirmation that you may be using.

There are many different techniques both for visualisation and for creating harmonious breathing, and, as with so many healing techniques, the important thing is to find the one which feels right for you.

You may find it helpful to imagine that you are lying under a large golden sun. Imagine – and feel – the warmth on your body; and as you breathe in, feel that you are breathing in the golden light of the sun. Imagine this light circulating through your bloodstream, healing and strengthening you. As you breathe out, you can either imagine the light reaching every organ of your body, or you can imagine that you are breathing out the sickness, pain, fear and so on, whichever feels most natural to you.

Or you might like to visualise yourself lying on a warm beach by the sea. As you breathe in, the waves come up and wash over you, healing and cleansing you; as you breathe out, they go back, taking your pain and sickness with them.

If you're not a particularly visual kind of person, you might prefer to say some words to yourself as you breathe in and out: 'love in', as you breathe in; and 'love out' as you breathe out; or just 'deep peace'; or any words or even syllables which feel harmonious to you.

Whichever method you use, after a while the breath is no longer just oxygen, but energy, and you can feel your body being energised and becoming warmer. Feel the energy flowing in and around your body and healing it. Feel it concentrating on the areas where you feel diseased; feel the energy flowing to that area and bringing love and healing. Gently tell the disease that it does not belong there any more; you might like to say to yourself 'I release the need for this disease.'

Some people like to use a cleansing visualisation, such as tiny brooms moving right through their system sweeping away the illness, or pointed arrows of light burning up diseased cells. See how it appears to you; trust your own ability to visualise or sense what is needed, and your body to respond and to heal itself. Try to feel a sense of love rather than of hate and anger towards the disease.

Accepting and Letting Go

Everyone responds to treatment in a unique way. It is important, therefore, to remain open and accepting. Try not to have preconceived ideas about different forms of treatment, how you 'should' respond, how quickly you 'should' get better, or the exact way in which your illness 'should' progress. It does not help to think of the disease as an enemy because healing is about wholeness, and while you feel that you and the disease are on opposite sides, you cannot be whole. The healing power within you will be able to flow if you let go of tension and resistance to your illness. Embrace the disease, whilst realising that it is not you; accept it fully as part of this life, whilst accepting too that you would prefer it to go.

Many people regard illness as a calamity and a punishment, and people who are ill are often ostracised; some diseases are not even talked about. But it is important for us to grow and to integrate all aspects of our being; illness is a painful teacher, but sometimes a very effective one. It also gives us a chance to withdraw from social activities in order to go within; then we can perhaps look at our own values and ask ourselves whether our lifestyle reflects these. Patients should not be viewed as 'sick people', but as people undergoing a particular transformation. Being close to people who are ill, and helping them, is one of the surest ways of rediscovering our own values.

Healing begins when you start to love yourself exactly as you are, at this moment, including your disease. You need to embrace yourself and your condition, whilst also accepting that you would like it to be different tomorrow . . . but that if it isn't, you will accept that too. Acceptance clears the space for the healing to take place. So open your eyes and see yourself as you really are, without criticism, accepting that 'This is how I am; this is the body I happen to be in; but I am not my body, or my mind, or my emotions, or my disease.'

In his book *Healing Into Life and Death*, Stephen Levine describes a technique which is helpful for relaxing and accepting yourself. He calls it 'soft belly'. You simply let your belly go, become rounded and relaxed, and see if that helps you to relax the tension in your body and accept yourself as you are, without holding in or worrying about appearances. Notice during the day how many times you tense your belly; each time relax it back to this state of 'soft belly', of acceptance, vulnerability, openness to healing. It will help if you wear loose, soft, comfortable clothes in natural fibres and colours which you love.

The choice we have is not whether we get better or remain sick; live or die; these things are out of our control. What we do have control over is the quality of our life in this moment. Concentrate on experiencing life now, fully, without allowing yourself to be troubled by regret about or yearning for the past, or expectations about the future. The reality is now; the past is gone, the future is yet to be, and may be totally different from how you fear, or imagine it will be. Letting go of both the past and the future removes the assumption that a disease you have had for ten years will be with you tomorrow; by letting go of expectation, you open the way for miracles of healing to occur.

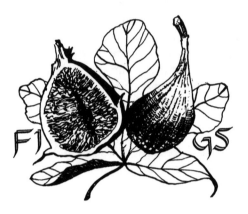

FIGS

Botanical Names of Tinctures and Herbs

Agrimony: *Agrimonia eupatoria*
Aloe: *Aloe vera*

Barberry: *Berberis vulgaris*
Bearberry: *Arctostaphylos uva-ursi*
Bistort: *Polygonum bistorta*
Blue Cohosh: *Caulophyllum thalictroides*
Boneset: *Eupatorium perfoliatum*
Borage: *Borago officinalis*
Buckthorn: *Rhamnus catharticus*
Bugleweed: *Lycopus virginicus*
Burdock: *Arctium lappa*

Camomile: *Matricaria recutita*
Capricin: *Capricin*
Cascara Sagrada: *Rhamnus purshiana*
Catmint: *Nepeta cataria*
Centaury: *Centaurium erythraea*
Chaparral: *Larrea tridentata*
Coltsfoot: *Tussilago farfara*
Comfrey: *Symphytum officinale*
Cornsilk (which comes from maize): *Zea mays*
Cramp bark (Guelder rose): *Viburnum opulus*
Cranesbill (American): *Geranium maculatum*

Dang Gui: *Angelica sinensis*
Devil's claw: *Harpagophytum procumbens*

Echinacea: *Echinacea angustifolia*
Elder flowers: *Sambucus nigra*
Elecampane: *Inula helenium*

Fennel: *Foeniculum vulgare*
Feverfew: *Chrysanthemum parthenium*
Figwort: *Scrophularia nodosa*

Ginger: *Zingiber officinale*
Ginseng, American: *Panax quinquefolius*
Ginseng, common: *Panax pseudoginseng*
Goat's rue: *Galega officinalis*
Golden-rod: *Solidago virgaurea*
Gou Qi Zi: *Licium chinese*
Guarana: *Paullinia cupana*

Hawthorn: *Crataegus oxyacantha*
Heartsease: *Viola tricolor*
Horsetail: *Equisetum arvense*
Huang chi: *Astragalus membranaceus*
Hypericum (St John's Wort): *Hypericum perforatum*

Jambul: *Syzygium jambolana*
Ju hua: *Chrysanthemum morifolium*

Lady's mantle: *Alchemilla vulgaris*
Lemon balm: *Melissa officinalis*
Lime flowers: *Tilia x europaea*
Liquorice: *Glycyrrhiza glabra*
Lobelia (Indian Tobacco): *Lobelia inflata*

Marigold: *Calendula officinalis*
Marigold, African: *Tagetes Ssp*
Marsh mallow: *Althaea officinalis*
Melilot: *Melilotus officinalis*
Mugwort: *Artemisia vulgaris*
Mullein: *Verbascum thapsus*

Nettle: *Urtica dioica*

Passion flower: *Passiflora incarnata*
Pellitory-of-the-wall: *Parietaria diffusa*
Plantain: *Plantago major*
Pokeroot: *Phytolacca decandra*
Psillium: *Plantago ovata*

Red clover: *Trifolium pratense*
Rehmania: *Rehmania glutinosae*
Reishi: *Ganoderna lucidum*

Shepherd's purse: *Capsella bursa-pastoris*
Skull-cap: *Scutellaria laterifolia*
Solidago (Golden-rod): *Solidago virgaurea*
Speedwell: *Veronica officinalis*

Violet: *Viola odorata*

Wu Wei Zi: *Schizandra*

Yarrow: *Achillea millefolium*
Yellow dock: *Rumex crispus*

The Remedies

COOL/COOLING

Herbs and spices
Lemon verbena
Mint
Rose
Rosehip
Hibiscus

Vegetables
Artichoke
Asparagus
Aubergine
Cabbage
Celery
Chicory, wild
Courgette
Cucumber
Dandelion
Fennel (bulb)
Lettuce
Radish
Seaweed
Spinach
Tomato

Grains
Barley
Millet
Wheat

Fruits
Apple
Banana
Bilberry
Blackcurrant
Fig
Grapefruit
Lemon
Lime
Melon
Orange
Peach
Pear
Pineapple
Pomegranate
Quince
Watermelon

NEUTRAL

Herbs and spices
Aniseed
Basil
Camomile
Coriander
Geranium
Lavender
Lemon thyme
Marigold
Marjoram
Parsley
Sage
Tarragon

Vegetables
Beetroot
Carrot
Pea
Potato

Pumpkin
Shiitake mushroom
Watercress

Pulses
Aduki bean
Broad bean
Chick pea
Haricot or Cannellini bean
Lentil
Miso
Mung bean
Dried pea
Red kidney bean
Soya bean
Tofu

Grains
Barley
Buckwheat
Maize
Brown rice
Rye

Nuts and seeds
Almond
Peanut
Sesame seed
Walnut

Fruits
Apricot
Avocado pear
Cherry
Date
Grape
Mandarin, tangerine
Mango
Pawpaw
Plum
Raspberry
Strawberry

WARM/WARMING

Herbs and spices
Bay leaf
Caraway
Cardamom
Cinnamon
Fennel (seed)
Nutmeg
Oregano

Vegetables
Nettle

Grains
Oats

Nuts and seeds
Chestnut
Pumpkin seed
Sunflower seed

HOT

Herbs and spices
Garlic
Ginger
Horseradish
Mustard
Chilli
Pepper
Savory
Thyme

Vegetables
Leek
Onion

Summary of Nutrients

THEIR SOURCES AND FUNCTIONS

Nutrient	Main Sources	Function
Protein	Milk; cheese; yogurt, eggs; legumes, including soya flour, tofu, and soya milk; nuts and seeds; cereals, wholegrain bread; wheatgerm	Growth and repair of body cells. Reproduction and formation of blood and bones. Protection against infection
Fibre	Legumes, nuts and seeds, wholegrain cereals, fresh and dried fruits, vegetables	Healthy functioning of the digestive system.
Fat	Oil, butter, margarine, whole milk, cream, yogurt, vegetable fats, egg yolk, cheese, nuts and seeds, avocado	Production of hormones and bile acids. Health of membranes. Polyunsaturated fats help absorption of vitamins A, D, and E. Source of energy.
Fat-Soluble Vitamins		
Vitamin A	Egg yolk, dairy products, fortified margarine, carrots, apricots, oranges, yellow and orange melons, peaches, mangoes, tomatoes, all green and some yellow vegetables.	Healthy eyes, skin, lungs, throat, hair, and nails. Increases resistance to infection. Helps in the healing process.

Nutrient	Main Sources	Function
Vitamin D	Butter, margarine, cottage cheese, yogurt, milk, evaporated milk, hard cheese, egg, action of sunlight on skin	Absorption of calcium for bones and teeth.
Vitamin E	Wholegrain cereals, wheatgerm, nuts, seeds, green leafy vegetables, legumes; cold-pressed vegetable oils (richest sources)	Improves general vitality and is important for proper functioning of the heart and cell structures
Vitamin K	Green leafy vegetables, soya bean oil, tomatoes, egg yolk, alfalfa	Blood clotting and prevention of excess loss of blood after injuries.

Water-Soluble Vitamins

Nutrient	Main Sources	Function
B Complex B1 Thiamin	Wholegrain bread, wheatgerm, fortified breakfast cereals, brewers' yeast, yeast extract, peanuts, brazil nuts, legumes, soya flour, oranges, dried egg yolk, dairy products	Involved in the release of energy from starch and sugars, and for the health of muscles, nerves, eyes, hair, skin, and blood.
B_2 (Riboflavin)	Fortified breakfast cereals, brewers' yeast, yeast extract, almonds, wheatgerm, dairy products, dark green leafy vegetables, mushrooms, potatoes, dried fruit, avocado, chocolate	Proper metabolism of starches and sugars, production of antibodies, and healthy function and development of the brain.

Nutrient	Main Sources	Function
Niacin	Fortified breakfast cereals, wheatgerm, wholegrain bread, milk and milk products, brewers' yeast, yeast extract, peanuts, almonds, leafy vegetables, mushrooms, avocado, chocolate, dried fruit (especially figs, apricots, prunes and peaches), legumes	Similar to riboflavin.
B_6 (Pyridoxine)	Brewers' yeast, yeast extract, wholegrain bread, wheatgerm, soya flour, walnuts, peanuts, legumes, eggs, milk, corn, sprouts, bananas	Utilisation of protein and production of haemoglobin.
Vitamin B_{12}	Dairy products, fortified foods, yeast extract	Similar to vitamins B_1, B_2, and niacin. Also for production of bone marrow.
Folic Acid	Wheatgerm, brewers' yeast, yeast extract, dark green leafy vegetables, raw peanuts and walnuts, raw cauliflower, mushrooms, tomatoes, oranges, potatoes, most fruit and vegetables, cow's milk (not goat's), eggs	Works with vitamin B_{12} in cell division. Vital in pregnancy.
Pantothenic Acid	Brewers' yeast, yeast extract, eggs, peanuts, wheatgerm, mushrooms, wholegrain bread and cereals, cheese, legumes	Release of energy from food. Proper functioning of adrenal glands.

Nutrient	Main Sources	Function
Vitamin C (Ascorbic Acid)	Oranges, grapefruit, strawberries, tomatoes, green leafy vegetables, potatoes, bean sprouts, red peppers	Increases resistance to infection. Helps in the healing process. Promotes normal growth.

Minerals

Nutrient	Main Sources	Function
Calcium	Milk, cheese, yogurt, legumes, sesame seeds, blackstrap molasses, sunflower seeds, almonds, green leafy vegetables (especially broccoli and spinach); carob, soya flour and milk, tofu, dried fruit (especially figs), brewers' yeast	Maintenance of healthy bones and teeth. Blood clotting. Healthy working of heart and skin.
Iron	Brewers' yeast, blackstrap molasses, legumes, soya flour and milk, tofu, green leafy vegetables, dried fruits, wholegrain bread and wholegrains, almonds, pumpkin seeds, eggs	Healthy blood. (Absorption aided by foods containing vitamin C.)
Magnesium	Wholegrains, wholegrain bread, wheatgerm, nuts (especially almonds, cashews, brazil nuts), legumes, soya flour, tofu, soya milk, brewers' yeast, fruit (especially bananas), vegetables (especially potatoes and leafy greens)	Release of energy from carbohydrates. Healthy formation of bones and teeth.

✑ Summary of Nutrients, Their Sources and Functions ☙

Nutrient	Main Sources	Function
Phosphorus	Usually present with calcium	Used with calcium for healthy bones and teeth
Potassium	In nearly all foods, especially vegetables, legumes, fruits, wholegrain bread, brewers' yeast, nuts, and seeds	Healthy cells, growth and health of the heart
Sodium	Table salt, sea salt, miso, tamari and shoyu soy sauce, celery, cheeses, nuts, egg yolk, dairy products	Many vital body functions.

Trace Elements

Zinc	Nuts, pumpkin seeds, dairy produce, eggs, brewers' yeast, legumes, peas, asparagus, spinach, cauliflower, mushrooms, mangoes, wholegrain bread, wholegrain cereals	Normal growth and healing.
Iodine	Seaweeds, including vegetarian jelling agents; soya beans, iodised salt, garlic, green vegetables	Needed by the thyroid gland.
Manganese	Wholegrain bread, wheatgerm, wholegrain cereals, nuts, dried figs, dates, peaches, apricots, brewers' yeast	Utilisation of vitamin B_1. Also needed in reproduction and lactation.

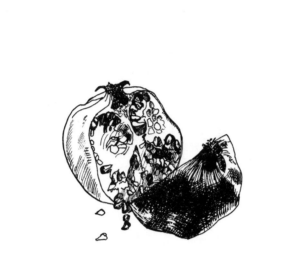

Bibliography and Further Reading

Bardeau, Fabrice, *Curarsi con i fiori*, Mondadori, Milan, 1976

Beeken, Jenny, *Yoga of the Heart*, The White Eagle Publishing Trust, 1990

Bensky, Dan, and Gamble, Andrew, *Chinese Herbal Medicine Materia Medica*, Eastland Press, Seattle, Oregon, 1986

Bouhours, Jack, *La salute del bambino con le piante*, Martello, Florence, 1982

Carpenter, Moira, *Curing P.M.T.: The Drug-free Way*, Arrow Books, 1985

Chaitow, Leon, *An End to Cancer?*, Thorsons, 1978

Chang, Dr Stephen, *The Complete System of Chinese Self-Healing*, The Aquarian Press, San Francisco, 1985

Chopra, Deepak, MD, *Quantum Healing*, Bantam Books, New York, 1989

Christopher, John, *School of Natural Healing*, Bi World, Provo, Utah, 1976

Culpeper's Complete Herbal, W. Foulsham & Co.

Davies, Patricia, *An A to Z of Aromatherapy*, The C.W. Daniel Co. Ltd, 1988

De Bairacli Levy, Juliette, *The Illustrated Herbal Handbook*, Faber, 1982

Dethlefson, T., and Dahlke, Dr R., *The Healing Power of Illness*, Element Books, Munich, 1983

Elliot, Rose, *Vegetarian Slimming*, Chapmans, 1991; *Rose Elliot's Mother and Baby Book*, Fontana, 1989; *Your Very Good Health*, Fontana, 1981

Garrison Jnr, Robert, and Somer, Elizabeth, *The Nutrition Desk Reference*, Keats Publishing, New Canaan, Connecticut, 1985

Gawain, Shakti, and King, Laurel, *Creative Visualisation*, Bantam Books, New York, 1987; *Living in the Light*, Eden Grove Publications, 1988

Grant, Doris, and Joice, Jean, *Don't Mix Foods Which Fight*, Thorsons, 1984

Gerard, *The Herbal*, Dover Press, Toronto, 1975

Grieve, M., *A Modern Herbal*, Penguin Books, 1931

Harrison, Dr John, *Love Your Disease, It Is Keeping You Healthy*, Angus & Robertson, 1985

Hay, Louise L., *You Can Heal Your Life*, Eden Grove Publications, 1988

Hertzka, Dr G., and Strehlow, Dr W., *Hildegard of Bingen's Medicine*, Bear & Co., Santa Fe, 1988

Hoare, Sophy, *Yoga*, Macdonald Guidelines, 1977

Howard, Judy, *The Back Flower Remedies Step by Step*, The C.W. Daniel Co. Ltd, 1990

Iyengar, B.K.S., *The Concise Light on Yoga*, Unwin Paperbacks, 1980

Jeffers, Susan, Ph.D., *Feel the Fear And Do It Anyway*, Ballantine Books, New York, 1987

LeShan, Laurence, *How to Meditate – A Guide to Self-Discovery*, Crucible, 1989

Levine, Stephen, *Who dies?*, Gateway Books, 1986; *Healing into Life and Death*, Gateway Books, 1989

Liu, Da, *T'ai Chi Ch'uan and Meditation*, Shocken Books, New York, 1986

Long, Ruth, *New Nutrition*, Keats Publishing, New Canaan, Connecticut, 1989

Lowen, Alexander, *The Way to Vibrant Health – a Manual of Bioenergetic Exercises*, Harper & Row, New York, 1977; *Bioenergetics*, Penguin Books, 1979

Lu, Henry, *Chinese System of Food Cures*, Sterling Publishing, New York, 1986

The Merck Manual, MSD, Rahway, New Jersey, 1899

Mervyn, Leonard, Ph.D., *The Dictionary of Vitamins and Minerals*, Thorsons, 1984

Nadkarni, Dr K., *Indian Materia Medica*, Popular Prakashan, Bombay, 1908

Ni, Maoshing, Ph.D., with McNease, Cathy, *The Tao of Nutrition*, College of Tao, Malibu, California, 1987

Paterson, Vicky, *Eat Your Way to Health*, Penguin Books, 1981

Reid, Daniel, *Chinese Herbal Medicine*, Thorsons, 1987

Scott, Julian, Ph.D., *Natural Medicine for Children*, Gaia, 1990

Shook, Dr Edward, *Advanced Treatise in Herbology*, Trinity Center Press, Beaumont, California, 1978

Shreeve, Dr Caroline, *The Alternative Dictionary of Symptoms and Cures*, Century, 1986

Soo, Chee, *The Chinese Art of T'ai Chi Ch'uan*, The Aquarian Press, 1984

Tisserand, Robert, *Aromatherapy*, Mayflower, 1977

Valnet, Dr Jean, *The Practice of Aromatherapy*, The C.W. Daniel Co. Ltd, 1982; *Cura delle malattiecon ortaggi, frutta e cerealo*, Giunti-Martello, Milan, 1975

Vaughan, Frances, *The Inward Arc*, New Science Library, 1986

Wu, K.K., *Therapeutic Breathing Exercise*, Hai Feng Publishing, Hong Kong, 1984

Yeoh, Aileen, *Longevity, the Tao of Eating and Healing*, Times Books Ltd, Singapore, 1989

Subject Index

Recipe Index